John

MW01206500

An overview of:

Cancer as a Metabolic Disease by Dr. Thomas Seyfried. On the Origin, Management, and Prevention of Cancer

———————

Including texts by Dominic D'Agostino and Travis Christofferson & the Press Pulse Strategy

———————

Revised Transcripts

(final revision of Chapter 1 - by Dr. Thomas Seyfried)

25% of the royalties will go to cancer research, via
The Foundation for Metabolic Cancer Therapies

————————————

ANY REVIEW WOULD BE GREATLY APPRECIATED TO GET THE MESSAGE OUT!

TABLE OF CONTENTS

Chapter 1

Dr. Thomas Seyfried:
Cancer as Metabolic Disease

Well, thank you very much. I'd like to thank CrossFit and Greg for supporting us. I'd also like to thank Jeff Glassman for the good questions that he asked us in the past, to validate some of our theories. You know, we need people like that, it's good to have people that question the information that you present. It makes us better at explaining this.

For your information: I have no financial disclosures.

Alright, So what I'd like to do to start this off is, basically, to present a report card on our approach to managing cancer.

And as I said, I'm going to speak to you today about cancer in general and also focus on specific types of cancer, in particular glioblastoma. As an illustrative example of our approach to managing the disease.

Now, these are numbers that we can take from the American Cancer Society, and they publish every year data on the overall number of cases and deaths. The war on cancer and the success that we're having is not going well.

So I compiled the data, just over the last five years:

Percentage increase for cancer deaths is greater than the increase for new cases!

Cancer Statistics in the U.S. from 2013-2017

Year	New Cases	Deaths/year	deaths/day
2013	1,660,290	580,350	1,590
2014	1,658,370	585,720	1,605
2015	1,658,370	589,430	1,615
2016	1,685,210	595,690	1,632
2017	1,688,780	600,920	1,646
% Increase	1,7%	3,4%	3,4%

Data from American Cancer Society

This is 2013 to 2017 and as you can see, these are pretty sobering numbers. We break them down into new cases, deaths per year and deaths per day, simply dividing by 365, to give an estimate. And you'll notice that the deaths per day and per year are exceeding that of the new cases. Not good.

Just to put things into perspective: The population increase in the United States over the same period of time was about 2.9 percent. So how is this war on cancer going? You look at the numbers, you can make your own decision. These are numbers you don't see on TV, right? You see Opdivo and Keytruda and that kind of stuff, but you don't see the constant increase in deaths per day.

So the question we have to ask ourselves is: What's going on here? We're not getting success here! This is a failure of monumental proportions, right? These are large numbers! In China it's over 8,000 a day dying from cancer. Cancer's already superseded heart disease in China!

We go out and we raise money for cancer, right? You all know, you run, jump... I don't know if you guys do 'CrossFit for cancer'. But everybody raises money for cancer, it makes them feel good. Nobody asks: How much of the money that we raise goes to cancer research? And what's more important: What kind of research are they doing with all that money?

The federal government's spending millions of dollars on cancer research. People are raising money, "Stand up to cancer!" Look, the more money we raise for cancer, the more cancer we get. So you have to say: What is going on here? How do you explain this?

And it has to do with a fundamental misunderstanding of what the nature of this disease is.

We've been led to believe, that this is a genetic disease and I'll present evidence to show that it's not.

Here's a simple cartoon of a cell with a nucleus and a mitochondrion, within a cell membrane:

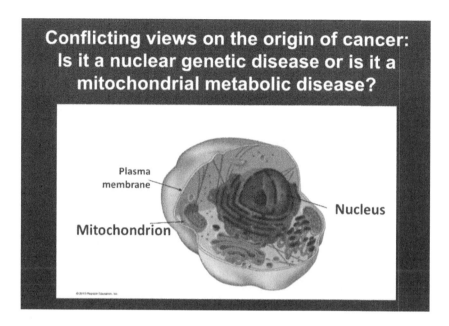

Conflicting views on the origin of cancer: Is it a nuclear genetic disease or is it a mitochondrial metabolic disease?

Plasma membrane

Nucleus

Mitochondrion

So we know there are mutations in the nucleus, but we also know that there are defects in the mitochondria as well. And I'll be showing you data showing that the origin of this disease is a mitochondrial metabolic abnormality. It's not a nuclear genetic disease. The mutations that you see in the nucleus are actually coming from reactive oxygen species (ROS) produced by the mitochondria!

What the entire field has been doing over the last six or seven decades, is chasing red herrings! Consequently, you have 1,600 people a day dying from the disease.

So the current dogma says: **Cancer is a genetic disease**. And this is solidified in this major paper:

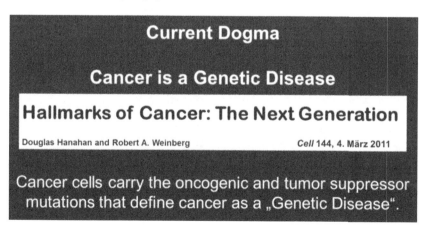

Current Dogma

Cancer is a Genetic Disease

Hallmarks of Cancer: The Next Generation

Douglas Hanahan and Robert A. Weinberg · *Cell* 144, 4. März 2011

Cancer cells carry the oncogenic and tumor suppressor mutations that define cancer as a „Genetic Disease".

Hallmarks of Cancer by Hanahan and Weinberg, one of the more highly cited papers in the entire cancer field. What they say is: Cancer cells carry the oncogenic and tumor suppressor mutations that define cancer as a genetic disease.

And we say it's a dogma, because it's presented as if it is an irrefutable truth. A dogma is no longer questioned, it's a solidified viewpoint. If you go into any textbook of biology, biochemistry or cell biology and you go to the cancer section, it says "cancer is a genetic disease." You go on to the NCI website, the National Cancer Institute, "cancer is a genetic disease."

There's no discussion about anything other than the fact that cancer is a genetic disease. Many of you went to medical school, you probably learned that cancer is a genetic disease. All the college courses on cell biology: Cancer is a genetic disease.

What this concept has done now, is it has indoctrinated several generations of scientists and physicians into this viewpoint that cancer is a genetic disease.

The somatic mutation theory is the foundation upon which the viewpoint of "cancer is a genetic disease" is based. And, basically, what the somatic mutation theory says, is that "Well, we get random mutations":

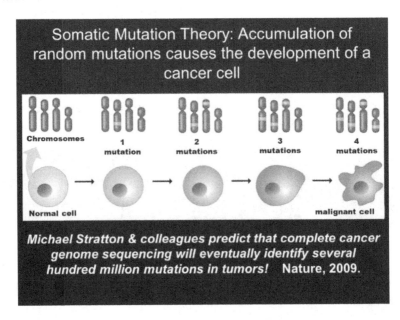

Somatic Mutation Theory: Accumulation of random mutations causes the development of a cancer cell

Chromosomes — 1 mutation — 2 mutations — 3 mutations — 4 mutations

Normal cell — malignant cell

Michael Stratton & colleagues predict that complete cancer genome sequencing will eventually identify several hundred million mutations in tumors! Nature, 2009.

<u>Random</u> mutations that accumulate. And eventually, you convert a normal appearing cell into this dysmorphic, mesenchymal kind of cell.

6

But nobody really knows how many mutations it takes to cause... or how it is related to the formation of a tumor. Is it 1, 2, or 4 mutations?

Michael Stratton from the UK says "We're going to have 100 million genes going to be found," and "look at the deep sequencing coming out of the Broad Institute," and these various places." Thousands and thousands of mutations have been identified.

And then they have to label them with different names, "drivers" and "passengers" and "go-alongs". A whole bunch of stuff is going on there.

And no one talks about those cancers that have no mutations! Kind of non-discussed.

So where does that all lead us to? Where have we come in this journey to manage cancer? We have now come to these terms "personalized therapy", "precision medicine"... all of this is based on the viewpoint that cancer is a genetic disease.

So you have these kinds of images, here:

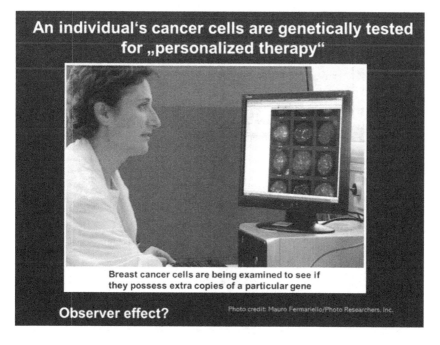

You have this woman staring into a screen and she's looking at breast cancer information to see if this may possess extra copies of a particular gene. Which would be used, in theory, as a diagnostic tool with possibly some therapeutic application. Now, to get that information usually you do needle biopsy.

So you have to take a needle biopsy of a particular tissue, in this case it would be a breast cancer. So you stab the tissue and in the process of stabbing the tissue, to get the information that she's looking at on that screen. Biopsy changes the micro environment of the tissue. You have potentially taken a pre-malignant state and by stabbing it to get this information, you have now put that person at risk.

Now, very interesting: The information that you get for this kind of screening is about $7,200 to do one of these screenings. To get the information that you can look at and say "Oh, we have this kind of battery of genes." Now, this would be okay if it had any redeeming value, right? But it has no value.

But you put people at risk for cancer by the very process of taking tissue. The phenomena is called inflammatory oncotaxis: It's an observer effect. By looking at it, you've changed it.

Now, I want to talk to you about the evidence that does not support the somatic mutation theory of cancer. And whenever you challenge any kind of a solidified dogma you always get the same response. We saw one of these images yesterday. This comes from Nikko, Japan. These are the Nikko monkeys:

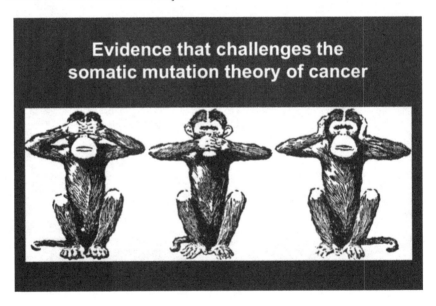

I went to japan, actually. They have carvings of them that are a little bit different than this, but it's basically similar: You don't want to look at the data, you don't want to talk about it, you don't want to hear about it. Anything that challenges your world view. I don't care if it's a religion, a political philosophy or a scientific concept. You generally get this kind of a response. I know it's hard, it's hard for people to look at things differently.

So what I did in chapter 11 of my book... This is a paper that I wrote a couple of years after the book, to update more and more of the issues associated with information that does not support the somatic mutation theory:

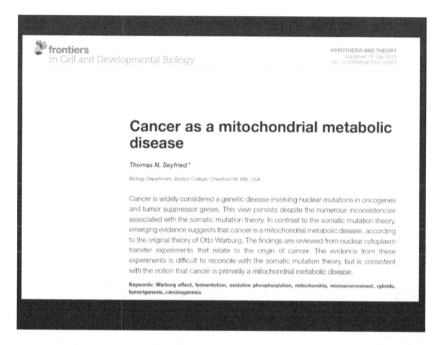

frontiers
in Cell and Developmental Biology

HYPOTHESIS AND THEORY
published: 07 July 2015
doi: 10.3389/fcell.2015.00043

Cancer as a mitochondrial metabolic disease

Thomas N. Seyfried *

Biology Department, Boston College, Chestnut Hill, MA, USA

Cancer is widely considered a genetic disease involving nuclear mutations in oncogenes and tumor suppressor genes. This view persists despite the numerous inconsistencies associated with the somatic mutation theory. In contrast to the somatic mutation theory, emerging evidence suggests that cancer is a mitochondrial metabolic disease, according to the original theory of Otto Warburg. The findings are reviewed from nuclear cytoplasm transfer experiments that relate to the origin of cancer. The evidence from these experiments is difficult to reconcile with the somatic mutation theory, but is consistent with the notion that cancer is primarily a mitochondrial metabolic disease.

Keywords: Warburg effect, fermentation, oxidative phosphorylation, mitochondria, microenvironment, cybrids, tumorigenesis, carcinogenesis

All I did was take articles from the literature that had been spattered about for years and brought them all together in one group of papers - and reevaluated the information from those papers in light of the two competing theories for the origin of the disease. So, bring them all together and then look at the data and then say "Do the data support more strongly one hypothesis, or theory, over the other?"

And you come to the conclusion that the somatic mutation theory makes no sense,- relative to the mitochondrial metabolic theory. You know, what's very interesting about this, when Gary gave his talk yesterday... about the difficulty in reproducing findings...

I find it remarkable that these different kinds of experiments were done by different individuals, with different tumor types, different protocols... but all coming to a similar conclusion that does not support the somatic mutation theory. But the data more strongly support Otto Warburg's theory of disturbed energy metabolism.

So let's just look at a couple of these experiments. And, you know, the important point about this paper is: Don't let anyone tell you what they think about it. You're smart people! I tell people "Read the original paper and you come to your own conclusion. You make your own decision." Don't ask "Hey, what do you think of that paper? Do you like it or not? Yeah, maybe it's no good".

You can't believe how many people take in information second, third hand, rather than going to the original source. Read it! You make your decision if you like it! Do what Dr. Glassman did, hit me with a thousand questions and I'll be happy to answer them!

So let's look at some of the data:

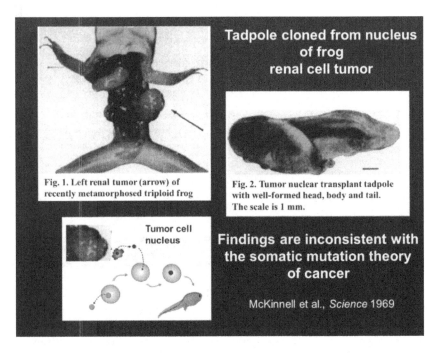

Tadpole cloned from nucleus of frog renal cell tumor

Fig. 1. Left renal tumor (arrow) of recently metamorphosed triploid frog

Fig. 2. Tumor nuclear transplant tadpole with well-formed head, body and tail. The scale is 1 mm.

Tumor cell nucleus

Findings are inconsistent with the somatic mutation theory of cancer

McKinnell et al., *Science* 1969

Now, this was done by McKinnell and his group, published in *Science* in 1969. I had the chance to speak with Dr. McKinnell before he passed away a couple years ago and we discussed these data at length.

So this frog has a massive renal tumor on the kidney. It's a kidney tumor, kills the frog, very aggressive. So what McKinnell and his group did is: They isolated cells from this kidney tumor and then they took the nucleus out of the kidney tumor cell and put it into a fertilized egg. The original nucleus of the egg was removed.

Here's the tumor cell, you take the nucleus that has the tumor suppressors and oncogenes and whatever - and you put it into this new cytoplasm that has normal mitochondria and you get a tadpole. And they looked very carefully, there was no evidence of the signature feature of cancer, dysregulated cell growth, anywhere. Everything looked perfectly normal.

The problem is, this tadpole could not fully develop into a mature frog. So whatever problem was in the tumor nucleus, it was not allowing the organism to fully mature. So the nuclear mutations didn't cause cancer, they blocked development.

These findings are inconsistent with the somatic mutation theory, which says, that the genes are causing the phenotype of dysregulated cell growth.

Another paper:

Reprogramming of a melanoma genome by nuclear transplantation

Konrad Hochedlinger,[1,4] Robert Blelloch,[1,2,4] Cameron Brennan,[3] Yasuhiro Yamada,[1] Minjung Kim,[3] Lynda Chin,[3,5] and Rudolf Jaenisch[1,6]

[1]Whitehead Institute for Biomedical Research, and Department of Biology, Massachusetts Institute of Technology, Cambridge, Massachusetts 02142, USA; [2]Department of Pathology, Brigham and Women's Hospital, Boston, Massachusetts 02115, USA; [3]Department of Medical Oncology, Dana-Farber Cancer Institute, Department of Dermatology, Harvard Medical School, Boston, Massachusetts 02115, USA

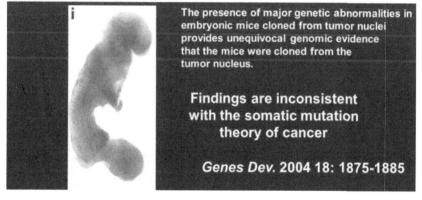

The presence of major genetic abnormalities in embryonic mice cloned from tumor nuclei provides unequivocal genomic evidence that the mice were cloned from the tumor nucleus.

Findings are inconsistent with the somatic mutation theory of cancer

Genes Dev. 2004 18: 1875-1885

I'm only going to give you information from a few of these studies, I put a whole bunch of these in the paper. It could take, you know, two days going over those experiments, but I'm just going to show you a few of them.

Now, this study was by Rudy Jaenisch and his colleagues at MIT. Rudy is one of the best and most preeminent developmental biologists. And he took these melanoma, malignant melanoma cells, and he characterized many of the mutations in the nucleus of the melanoma cell. They then he took the nucleus and made embryonic stem cells and cloned mice from the nucleus of melanomas.

He says here "The presence of major genetic abnormalities in embryonic mice cloned from the tumor nuclei provides unequivocal genomic evidence, that the mice were cloned from the tumor nucleus" - but they did not show any dysregulated cell growth. These findings are inconsistent with the somatic mutation theory of cancer.

And there was another series of experiments that were done by Dr. Wong and her group at Baylor College of Medicine, where they swapped the mitochondria from one cell to the next. These are much more difficult experiments than the nuclear transfer experiments.

So they take aggressive, malignant metastatic breast cancer cells, remove the mitochondria from the cytoplasm and bring in normal mitochondria from normal cells that don't have cancer. And the oncogenes and the abnormal growth was suppressed.

On the other hand, they took the mitochondria from the aggressive breast cancer cells and put them into an indolent cell (a type of low growth cancer) they exploded into high growth. So you've got a very different result. The mitochondria are calling the shots, not the nucleus!

So what we did to convey and summarize all of these data from all of these kinds of nuclear/mitochondrial transfer experiments in this simple diagram, which is now making its way through the web:

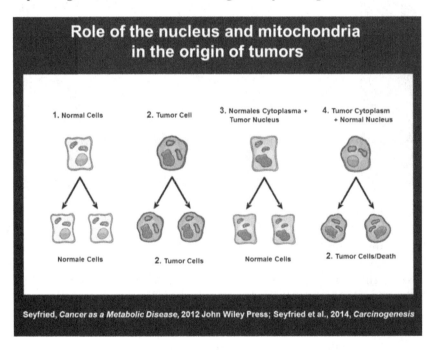

What I show here is: The green cell, which is a normal cell, begets normal cells. They have a normal genome, they have normal respiration. The red cell is the tumor cell. Tumor cells beget tumor cells. One tumor cell begets more tumor cells. They have genetic defects in the nucleus and they also have defects in the mitochondria.

Now, what is the origin of the disease? Is it the defects in the nucleus or is it the defects in the mitochondria? The nuclear transfer and mitochondrial transfer experiments provide evidence for this: Take the red nucleus and move it into the green cytoplasm - and you get normal cells that behave normally, grow normally, form normal tissues, sometimes organs and sometimes whole mice or frogs.

On the other hand Israel and Schaefer took the green nucleus and put it into the red cytoplasm. And in that case, you got either dead cells or tumor cells. You did not get normal cells. These are the exact opposite findings you would expect if the disease were a genetic disease!

Nuclear/mitochondrial transfer experiments are the strongest evidence to date that undermines the gene theory of cancer. The strongest evidence. No one has yet been able to explain how we get all these findings based on the somatic mutation theory of cancer!

So if that's the case: Why is the oncology field continuing to persist with therapies that are based on a flawed underlying hypothesis?

If somatic mutations are not the origin of cancer, how do we get cancer cells?

Well, Otto Warburg described this a long time ago, back in the early part of the 20th century:

On the Origin of Cancer Cells
Otto Warburg (Science, 24 February, 1956)

Warburg Theory of Cancer

1. Cancer arises from damage to cellular respiration.

2. Energy through fermentation gradually compensates for insufficient respiration.

3. Cancer cells continue to ferment lactate in the presence of oxygen (Warburg effect).

4. Enhanced fermentation is the signature metabolic malady of all cancer cells.

- Cancer cells arise from damage to the respiration
- Energy through fermentation gradually compensates for the insufficient respiration
- Cancer cells continue to ferment lactic acid in the presence of oxygen

This is called the "Warburg Effect" and unfortunately the Warburg Effect has significantly confused this field, making it confusing to a lot of people. Because they said "Well, there's some tumor cells that don't show a Warburg Effect, therefore Otto Warburg must be wrong!"

Well, myself and some of my colleagues, we proposed that cancer cells can not only ferment sugar (glucose), but they can also ferment amino acids. And that amino acid is primarily glutamine, through the succinyl-CoA-ligase step and this is not well known to a lot of people. Basically, this is the missing link in Warburg's central theory.

So the cells are fermenting, but not only lactic acid, they can ferment amino acids and particularly glutamine. I'll present evidence for that.

- Enhanced fermentation is the signature metabolic malady of all cancer cells

Now, if we take a tumor and we look at this tumor and we separate the cells of the tumor: Every single cell in that tumor has a different genetic profile. No two cells in that tumor have the same kinds of mutations! This has been demonstrated over and over again.

However, every cell in that tumor is fermenting. Now, the question I ask to you: Is it more logical to focus on the common problem that exists in all of the cells of the tumor - or do you think it makes more sense to focus on the individual, unique differences of every cell in that tumor? Right? I mean, the answer should be clear.

But we do it wrong! We focus on the unique, individual differences at the expense of the common pathophysiology - and that's what we call the somatic mutation theory of cancer. Consequently, we get 1,600 people dying a day.

Now, let's look at this, energy:

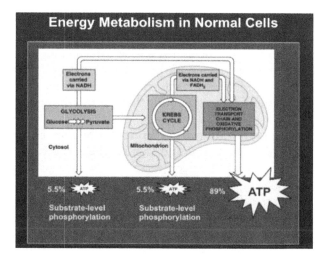

Alright. So, in a normal situation (this is a cartoon of just the mitochondria) most of the energy that we get in our body comes from breathing. About 89 to 90 percent through oxidative phosphorylation, respiration. We get smaller amounts of energy through these ancient pathways of substrate-level phosphorylation. In the cytoplasm, in the form of glycolysis and in the mitochondrial Krebs cycle through the succinyl-CoA-ligase step.

And we all know this, this is biochemistry, right? We're all breathing! We all are... well, I think. Any zombies out here? They don't breathe. But the issue is: Most of us breathe and when you exercise you breathe more and this is where we get our energy from, right?

Okay, now look at the cancer cell:

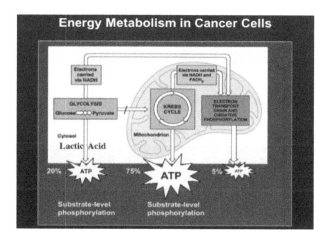

15

This is the same picture, but you'll notice that there's a major shift in where the energy is coming from. Much less energy is coming out of oxidative phosphorylation and a lot more is coming from these ancient, primitive pathways: substrate level phosphorylation.

And you see that... we now know, and we're learning more, that the majority of the energy is coming out of the mitochondria, but not through OxPhos [oxidative phosphorylation], but through the Krebs cycle. This is the new understanding that we're talking about, this is the missing link in Warburg's theory.

So tumors get a lot of energy from fermentation metabolism. Tumors can get energy without oxygen and this is where the cancer cells are getting their energy from! So people say "How do we get cancer then?" Well, all we have to do is take all of the data that was published in the cancer field over the last, you know, 100 years and just reconfigure it, along with Hanahan and Weinberg's *Hallmarks* paper.

Then we take the information and just rearrange the picture. And now we can put together, in a more logical way, the origin of "How we get cancer" - and once we know that, then we'll know how to manage the disease. It becomes much more clear to do that:

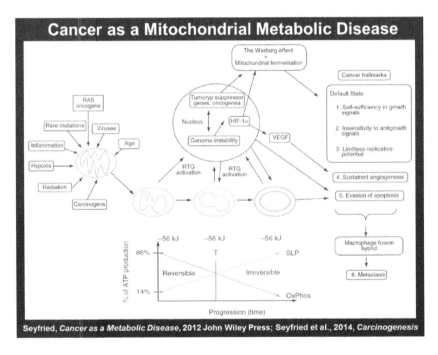

Cancer as a Mitochondrial Metabolic Disease

Seyfried, *Cancer as a Metabolic Disease*, 2012 John Wiley Press; Seyfried et al., 2014, *Carcinogenesis*

So what we have here on the on the left is the mitochondrion and people say "How do you get cancer?" Well, you can get cancer from any number of different things, right? Carcinogens cause cancer. You can get cancer if you're exposed to carcinogens. Radiation will cause cancer. Hypoxia (absence of oxygen) can cause cancer. Systemic inflammation, we heard that from Axel, he was telling us about the systemic inflammation and others.

Rare inherited mutations: People say "It must be genetic, because you got BRCA1 and P53... Angelina Jolie had her breasts and ovaries removed because of the BRCA1, she's trying to reduce her risk...

That's all secondary. It's secondary, because those BRCA1-mutations do not cause cancer, unless it damages the respiration. And there are people around that have BRCA1s who'll never get cancer, because the gene is not damaging the respiration.

Ras oncogene damages respiration.

Hepatitis C, and papilloma viruses enter mitochondria and damage the respiration. Age increases risk for cancer... so all these disparate risks factors was referred to as the oncogenic paradox, right?

Oncogenic Paradox

This was first pointed out by Albert Szent-Györgyi, who said "Hey, there's so many different ways to get cancer - but the common pathophysiological mechanism is not clear!" Well, once you understand that it's a mitochondrial metabolic disease, the mechanism becomes very clear!

And if you read Sid Mukherjee's book on the *Emperor of all maladies*, the one that was on the New York Times bestseller list, and it was the Pulitzer Prize-winning book on cancer... he struggles with this! If you read pages 285 and 303 in his book, he says "You know, it's just like, we don't... we just can't figure out how you get cancer from all these different things!"

You get cancer from all these different things, because they damage respiration and they form reactive oxygen species [ROS]. And reactive oxygen species are carcinogenic and mutagenic!

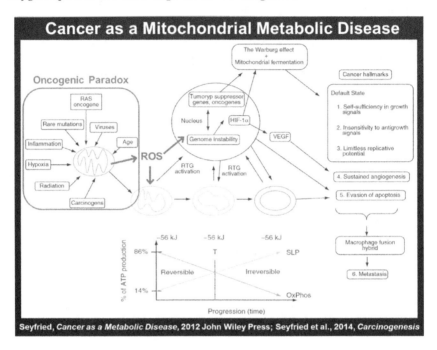

Cancer as a Mitochondrial Metabolic Disease

Seyfried, *Cancer as a Metabolic Disease*, 2012 John Wiley Press; Seyfried et al., 2014, *Carcinogenesis*

So the mutations that you see in the nucleus, that everybody is following - these red herrings - are all coming as a secondary cause to the damage to the respiration.

They are not the cause, they are the effects!

Alright? And then when the ROS are generated, they damage further the respiration, the cells are suffocating! Where are they going to get their energy? They have to upregulate substrate level phosphorylation.

So you see here at the bottom, the green line going down and the red line going up, substrate level phosphorylation. Which means a fermentation metabolism. So what are they fermenting? They're fermenting glucose and glutamine! Those are the two fuels that are driving up the energy. Because without energy nothing lives! Period!

Energy is everything. Without energy, you don't survive!

So what's happening with these cells is: They're shifting their energy away from respiration to a fermentation metabolism, using available fermentable fuels. So now we can put together all of the hallmarks of cancer in a more logical way, all linked back to damage to the respiration.

The first three hallmarks of Hanahan and Weinberg are all the result of the cell falling back on its default state, the state that the cells had before oxygen came into the atmosphere, some 2.5 billion years ago! Where everything on the planet was fermenting. They were fermenting amino acids and whatever else they can get!

And during that period of time the cells were in a state of unbridled proliferation and they would proliferate like crazy, until the fermentable fuels in the micro environment disappeared and they croaked. And they'd throw out all this waste material into the micro environment. In cancer this leads to vascularization or angiogenesis - another multi-billion dollar industry that's all based on, you know, indirect findings.

Okay. Then you say "Well, if this cancer cell is starting to suffocate, it should die, right?" Yeah, it should undergo programmed cell death and drop dead, that's called apoptosis. Why are they not undergoing apoptosis? Because the mitochondria control the apoptotic signaling system in the cell. Mitochondria are the cell's 'kill switch'! And your kill switch is broken and these cells are now bypassing apoptosis. They're not dying, they're proliferating.

So the big dog in this whole thing is metastasis. Okay, you know, I can agree with this. Where do you get metastasis from? Which is ultimately the biggest challenge in managing cancers, trying to control when it spreads through your body.

Now, you have to understand the biology of the disease. Once you understand the biology of the disease, you can start putting the pieces of the puzzle together:

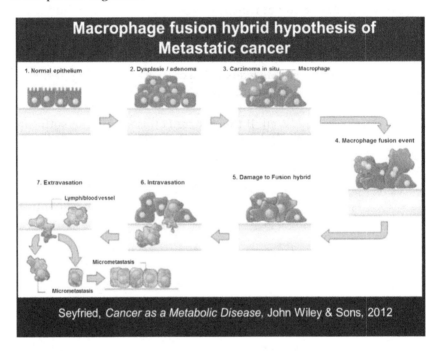

Seyfried, *Cancer as a Metabolic Disease*, John Wiley & Sons, 2012

Here's some blue cells, they're columnar epithelial cells. They could be in the breast, the colon or whatever. They get damaged by anyone of the provocative agents in the micro environment. They start entering the default state, they start proliferating.

Our body has a sensory system to know what's going on, this looks like an unhealed wound. So we have cells in our immune system that come into these places to heal wounds. And these are mostly macrophages. So they sense this, chemically, in the blood. They come in, out of the bloodstream, and they go right to these incipient cancer cells, growths of cells, to put out the fire, to heal the wound and then heal the tissue.

The problem is they throw out growth factors and cytokines, which are actually stimulatory towards these cells, which lost their growth control because of their fermentation behavior.

Now, they're making the situation worse, because it's the wrong context. What these red cells, our immune cells, do is to facilitate wound healing. They fuse together – they are very fusogenic cells, which is well documented in the scientific literature. So what's happening then with this continual fusion in this inflamed micro environment, is: You're diluting the cytoplasm of the red cell with the cytoplasm of the tumor cell, thereby shifting the immune cells from a respiratory system to a fermentation system, locked in.

These immune cells are already genetically programmed to enter and exit the bloodstream. You don't have to have this epithelial–mesenchymal transition, it makes absolutely no sense. (This is the gene theory explanation for metastasis.) This is the real thing! And we have evidence to support that in a number of different ways.

So you now have a rogue cell, part of our immune system, that's already programmed to spread through your body. Very difficult, they're already programmed to live in hypoxic environments, therefore anti-angiogenic drugs probably won't work - and they haven't worked.

So we now know the biology of the metastatic cell: It's a rogue macrophage! What do they eat? They eat glucose and glutamine! Okay. We know that.

Now, if most cancer cells obtain energy through fermentation, what therapies might be effective in managing tumors?

Well, one of the things, logically, is simply take away fermentable fuels and replace them in the body with non-fermentable fuels. And one of the ways to do that is: Stop eating! Calorie restriction [CR], ketogenic diets [KD], these kinds of things!

Calorie Restriction (CR) and Ketogenic Diets: A Metabolic Cancer Intervention

- CR involves a total dietary restriction

- CR differs from starvation

- CR maintains minerals and nutrients

- CR & KD reduce blood glucose and elevate ketone bodies, a non-fermentable fuel.

- CR & KD enhance mitochondrial biogenesis & OxPhos

- CR in mice equates to water-only fasting in humans

What calorie restriction and ketogenic diets do is:
- they differ from starvation
- they maintain normal levels of minerals
- they enhance mitochondrial biogenesis, and also, they replace fermentable fuels

You can't ferment ketone bodies! You need good respiration to obtain energy from ketone bodies. So you're going to remove or lower the glucose levels, and raise the ketone bodies which the normal cells are going to shift over to and the tumor cells are going to be marginalized because they can't use the ketone bodies!

And don't forget: We just heard from Michael about the basal metabolic rate. I do this in the mice. The mice, we give them 40% calorie restriction [CR] - but that's like water only fasting in humans, okay? People have to have to realize that because of the 7-fold difference in basal metabolic rate between mouse and human.

So ketogenic diets:

Composition (%) of the standard diet (SD) and the ketogenic diet (KD)

Components	Standard Diet (SD)	Ketogenic Diet (KD)
Carbohydrate	62	3
Fat	6	72
Protein	27	15
Energy (Kcal/gr)	4,4	7,2
F/ (P + C)	0,07	4

* The ketogenic diet should always be consumed in restricted amounts!

A lot of misinformation, a lot of misunderstanding. Basically, these are low-carb diets, high-fat diets. But it's the types of fats and proteins that play an important role.

Basically, you eat these diets in a restricted amount. The ketogenic diet, unfortunately it was labeled with the word 'diet', right? Whenever you put 'diet' on something, everything becomes like mysterious. It's a medicine! The ketogenic diet is a medicine, it's called *ketogenic metabolic therapy* and it should be respected as a medicine! If it's not used properly, it won't work, just like any medicine.

Not to say that it will harm you, but if you do eat too much ketogenic diet, you can in fact get insulin insensitivity. We worked in the epilepsy field for years and we understand how some of these diets can be not as effective as they should be.

But the whole strategy is not complicated, right? If the tumor cell needs fermentable fuel, then you take the fermentable fuel away from the tumor cell and you transition the body to a non-fermentable status:

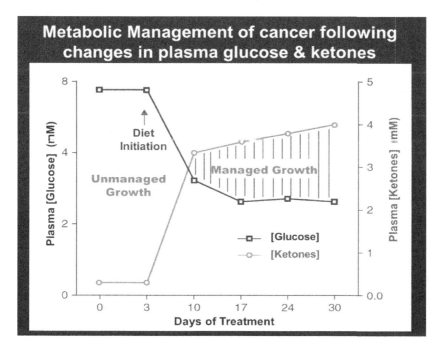

So you lower the blood sugar that the tumor cells need and you elevate ketone bodies, which the tumor cells can't use - but the normal cells can. You just simply marginalize the tumor.

Now, the tumor needs fuel, it can't live without energy. Where is it getting its fuel? It's fermenting. You're taking away a prime fuel - what's going to happen to those tumor cells? They're either going to die or they're going to slow down. And that's what happens!

Now, the first person that did this work was Linda Nebling, in a human situation, I should say:

Effects of a Ketogenic Diet on Tumor Metabolism and Nutritional Status in Pediatric Oncology Patients: Two Case Reports

Linda C. Nebling, PhD, MPH, RD, Floro Miraldi, MD, PhD, Susan B. Shurin, MD, and Edith Lerner, PhD, LD, FACN

Journal of the American College of Nutrition, Vol. 14, No. 2, 202–208 (1995)

The results showed that a ketogenic diet, which reduced blood glucose and elevated blood ketones, could provide long-term management in two children with recurrent inoperable brain tumors.

She took two little children, hopeless cases. Brutalized. Brutalized by the system. If you read her PhD dissertation, you'd be crushed about what they did to these little kids. They surgically mutilated them, gave them massive doses of chemo, radiation, all kinds of stuff. And they gave them up for hopeless, they said these kids aren't going to live more than two or three months.

She says "Can I try a ketogenic diet?" She was in nursing, getting her PhD in nursing. "Yeah, it's not going to do anything, they don't have long to live". So anyway, she rescued both of these kids! Their quality of life improved dramatically, they lived far longer than what was predicted. And it was based on the whole shift of the body's metabolism and I said "Wow, this is unbelievable!"

This was back in 1995 and I said to my students "You know, we should try some of that with our brain cancer and the mice!" And we were building these animal models, beautiful animal models of human brain cancers and we had the CT-2A, a neural stem cell tumor. Everybody's excited about neural stem cell cancers.

Anyway, we just gave them a standard diet [SD] - which is a high carb diet - but calorie restricted by 40%. Which is like a water-only therapeutic fast in humans:

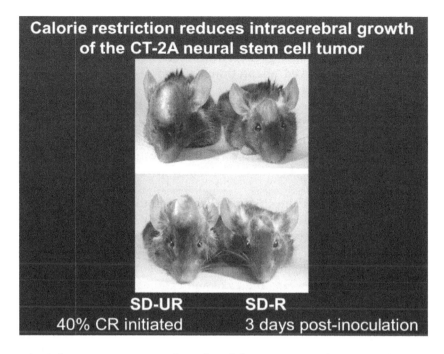

Calorie restriction reduces intracerebral growth of the CT-2A neural stem cell tumor

SD-UR SD-R
40% CR initiated 3 days post-inoculation

And these tumors started to shrink big time! You know, go down 60 to 85 percent reduction in size.

And we said "Geez, what? Wow!" You know, I never saw anything like this before, so powerful, "What's going on?"

So then we analyzed, using linear regression analysis, using glucose as the independent variable, and either ketones or tumor weight as the dependent variables and glucose as the independent:

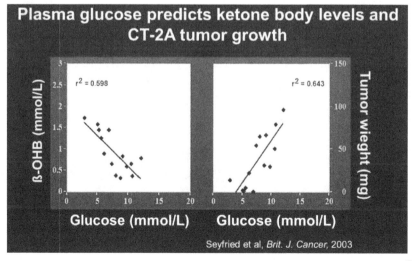

Plasma glucose predicts ketone body levels and CT-2A tumor growth

$r^2 = 0.598$ $r^2 = 0.643$

ß-OHB (mmol/L) Tumor wieght (mg)

Glucose (mmol/L) Glucose (mmol/L)

Seyfried et al, *Brit. J. Cancer*, 2003

Each square is an animal on a different diet. And you can see on the left here: As blood sugar goes down, ketones go up. And this is an evolutionarily conserved adaptation to food restriction. When our bodies are not getting the carbs, we're going to start mobilizing fats, bring them to the liver, chop them up, make water-soluble ketone bodies and these are going to go to the the the tissues.

And on the right side: The blood sugar goes down, the size of the tumor goes down. The higher the sugar, the faster the tumor grows - the lower the glucose, the slower the tumor grows! Right?

So the higher the sugar, the faster your tumor grows.
The lower the sugar, the slower your tumor grows.

So if you want your tumor to grow fast, get your blood sugar up as high as it can get! Right? You go to oncology clinics and you see everybody eating ice cream and cake and candies! Don't they read the literature? This has been supported now in human gliomas, breast cancer, colon cancer... if you want your tumor to grow fast, get the sugar as high as it can go!

Now people say "Well, this looks wonderful and great, but we don't understand the mechanism." Bullshit! You understand the mechanism! We published so many papers and so many other people published papers on the mechanisms by which this works!

Calorie Restriction & KD Target Major Cancer Hallmarks

1. **Anti-angiogenic**
   Mukherjee et al., Clin. Cancer Res., 2004

2. **Anti-inflammatory**
   Mulrooney et al., PLOS One, 2011

3. **Pro-apoptotic**
   Mukherjee et al., Brit. J. Cancer 2002

It's anti-angiogenic, anti-inflammatory, pro-apoptotic. No cancer drug is known that can do this without toxicity! And therapeutic fasting can do it! So we and others have shown in many papers the molecular mechanisms by which this process works.

When you hear people say "Well, it's not proven!" – Well, they don't read the literature, nor do they contribute to it!

So this woman had this dog with a big mast tumor on his nose, right? Minka. You know, she listens to our YouTube videos and reads our regular papers. She's a lay person, doesn't have any training in medicine or anything.

This dog has this big tumor, she goes to the vet, who said "Well, yeah we're going to have to cut it out and then we're going to give radiation and chemo. 'about ten thousand dollars, maybe the dog will live seven more months. But it's going to be sick..." and blah blah, you know. The same stuff.

She said no. So she went to the butcher and she got the fresh chicken meat with the bones in it. Cut the calories by 40 percent, threw in some medium chain triglyceride [MCT] oil and some raw eggs in the mix. The dog lost about five percent of its body weight.

And you can see: The tumor started to shrink and disappear!

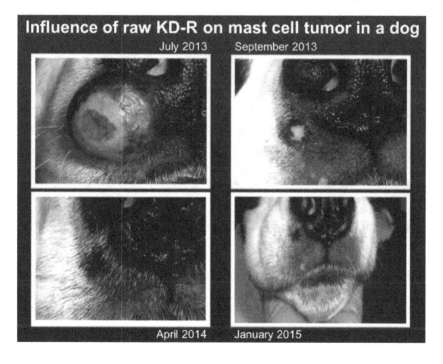

Influence of raw KD-R on mast cell tumor in a dog
July 2013   September 2013
April 2014   January 2015

And, you know, Minka is still alive today, doing fine! This was back in 2013. Impressive, how fast the dog responded, and there's many dogs now. They're putting them through these metabolic therapies that are doing really well.

Of course, the veterinarians were all over me about this. They don't think they should feed the raw meat to the dogs because of salmonella poisoning! Give me a break! I mean... have you ever seen what dogs eat? It's like, give me a break, you know! Salmonella poisoning!

So you're looking at this stuff and you're saying "Jesus!"... and then we did a YouTube video on this, about the dog cancer thing, got 5.3 million hits! Can you believe this? So there were all kinds of trolls out there, writing all these negative reports, giving me all kinds of grief. The hell with them, you know.

Okay. Now I want to talk about a really serious issue here, glioblastoma multiforme. And this is a really bad tumor with poor prognosis:

Glioblastoma Multiforme

- Among the most aggressive of all primary brain tumors

- Poor prognosis

- No effective therapies

- Composed of multiple cell types:
  Neoplastic Stem cells
  Neoplastic mesenchymal migroglia

- Highly Invasive, „Secondary Structures of Scherer"

- Metastatic outside the CNS

And unfortunately Senator John McCain is now struggling with this kind of a tumor. It's a nasty cancer, many multiple different kinds of cells, no effective therapy. So you get a whole bunch of different kinds of cells. Consequently the name "multiforme": Highly invasive.

So when you look at a brain tumor... here's a poor soul that sacrificed their brain for the study. And you can see: This nasty necrotic area, a cyst, large cyst:

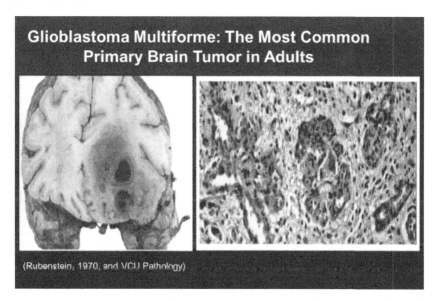

Glioblastoma Multiforme: The Most Common Primary Brain Tumor in Adults

(Rubenstein, 1970, and VCU Pathology)

But, if you look at the midline of the brain, you can see it shifted to the left. This is called "midline shift", okay?

So these tumors grow and they cause intercranial pressure. And people die from intracranial pressure, most of the people who have these kinds of tumors. The problem is: You can't surgically resect them, because the tumor cells have already spread out into the normal appearing brain areas. And the tumor cells use blood vessels as one of the mechanisms to disseminate: They go across the surface of blood vessels in the Virchow-Robin space.

So they use these blood vessels as kind of a railroad system to get through the brain. So it's very, very hard to do any kind of surgical resection. And you can see them, the dark blue cells around the blood vessels are the way... you can see on histology. Histology will tell you. This is how they spread through the brain and make it very difficult to get resolution.

And we all know that mitochondria are abnormal in brain cancer.

This picture shows an electron micrograph... the only way you can see mitochondria clearly is EM, electron microscopy:

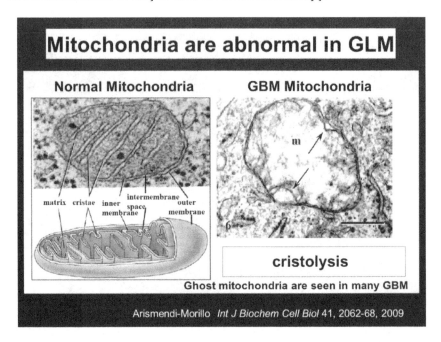

Mitochondria are abnormal in GLM

Normal Mitochondria | GBM Mitochondria

cristolysis

Ghost mitochondria are seen in many GBM

Arismendi-Morillo *Int J Biochem Cell Biol* 41, 2062-68, 2009

And the stripes in the mitochondria contain the proteins and the lipids of the electron transport chain, that allow us to get energy through oxidative phosphorylation. So you can see the nice stripes on the normal mitochondria there on the left. And the cristae are missing in GBM mitochondria, This is called cristolysis. The structure... the very structure of the organelle needed for oxidative phosphorylation is missing!!

Anybody can see the emptiness in that mitochondria. The stripes are missing! The stripes are missing, therefore the oxidative phosphorylation is missing, therefore the cell must ferment in order to survive. Everybody see that? Okay. There's a lot of papers in the literature showing that - yet, many members of my field say "The Mitochondria are normal". They obviously don't look at this or they don't want to see it.

The tumor cells ferment! They have to ferment, they don't have the structure. Structure dictates function. Without the structure, you can't get the function. The function is abnormal, because the structure is abnormal and my colleague Gabriel Arismendi-Morillo has published many beautiful papers on this.

So, if you can't get energy from oxidative phosphorylation, where do you get the energy to drive the beast? Where is that energy coming from? It's coming from glucose and glutamine - the two prime fuels that are going to drive the beast! They can't eat anything else! It's not there in sufficient quantity, we did the logistics on this.

These two fuels are abundant in the micro environment. So they come in, right? The two fuels together are synergistic:

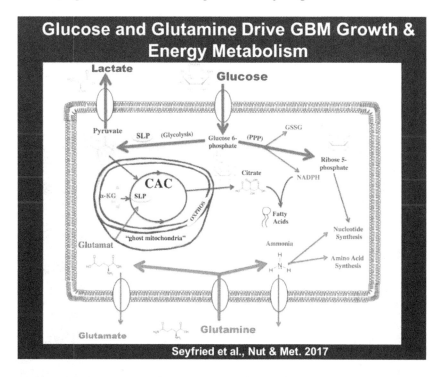

Glucose, glutamine. They come in, they fire the glycolytic pathway, the pentose pathway, the glutaminolysis pathway, deriving energy from substrate level phosphorylation. Making all of the stuff, the DNA-RNA proliferation... these cells grow like crazy.

So, what do we do in the clinic? Okay, so some poor soul comes in, diagnosed with a glioblastoma, devastating, you know. People don't know what they're going to do, you're just devastated. The patient's devastated, the family is devastated.

It's "My god, what's going on here?" - "Well, we have to do surgery, cut that tumor out right away!"

Sometimes you have to do that, when there's a herniation problem. But many times, you don't! You have a watchful waiting period. "No, no, no, we get them in as quickly as possible. We're going to debulk the tumor."

Surgeon takes out the tumor. Patient's sitting there, wakes up, "Oh, wow."

"Hey, how do you feel?"

"I feel pretty good."

"Okay. Now, as soon as you've recovered we're going to start giving you radiation therapy!"

So in the brain neurons and glia have a very close connection with each other. Intimate relationship, right? It's called the glutamine-glutamate cycle. It keeps our neurotransmitters in balance and everything is under control.

You break that glutamine-glutamate cycle, this happens:

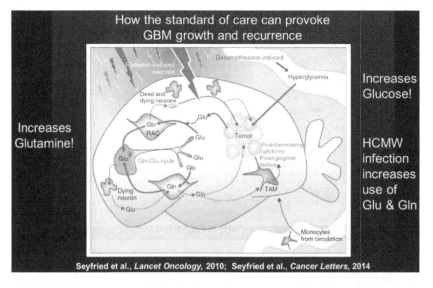

Glutamate (which is an excitatory neurotransmitter) comes out, excites neurons, they die, you get necrotic death. Astrocytes take up the glutamate, turn it into glutamine.

Now, those tumor cells that have not been debulked will now sucking down the glutamine, created by not only the wound from the surgeon, but also by the radiation that's blowing the hell out of the micro environment in this tumor. Creating a vast amount of glutamine, which is one of the powerful fuels driving the beast, as I just said!

Now, when you take somebody and surgically resect the bulk of the tumor and then start radiating their brain, you start to get head swelling, brain swelling, from the radiation. Causing the heat, the edema. To reduce the edema we give them high dose steroids. High dose steroids create hyperglycemia! Right? Glucose! Glucose and glutamine are now created by the very procedures that are used to treat the patient!

To make matters worse, 90 percent of the brain tumor cells are infected with human cytomegalovirus, which is a supercharger for allowing the tumor cells to use glucose and glutamine!

I published this paper in *Lancet Oncology,* saying that the standard of care contributes to the growth and the recurrence of the tumor! Based on hard biochemical evidence! What do you think the response was? They don't want to hear about it!

Now, let's test the hypothesis about what I just said, okay?

Look at the results from treating patients with brain tumors with the standard of care:

GBM Patient Survival under current „Standard of Care"

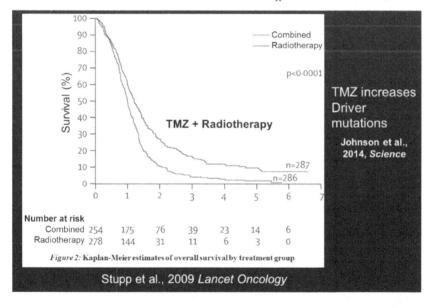

Figure 2: Kaplan-Meier estimates of overall survival by treatment group

Stupp et al., 2009 *Lancet Oncology*

So we have two lines here: The red line are those individuals that got radiation alone - and the blue line of those individuals who got radiation coupled with the toxic alkylating agent called Temozolomide [TMZ]. The fact that Temozolomide could contribute a little bit to survival was the single greatest advance in glioblastoma management in the last 50 years! Can you believe this? I was there, when they said this.

Now, look at the red line, the bottom line: The guys that got the radiation alone. How many survivors came out of the study? What's that number down at the end there? Zero! This has been reproduced. You want to know about replicating data? This has been reproduced in every country in the world, over and over again. Nothing is more certain than irradiating people and having them all dead!

Now we throw in TMZ. "But hey, listen! TMZ is doing something!" Well, you get a few extra survivors from this. So, I said to myself and my students "What does TMZ do?" So we looked and we found out, the adverse effects of temozolomide are: Diarrhea, vomiting, nausea and fatigue. Wow! These are all indirect forms of calorie restriction!

So, we published and we said that we think that blip in survival rate is due to indirect calorie restriction. Do you think anybody ran out to test that hypothesis? No!

You know, Temozolomide also increases driver mutations. What the hell does that mean? Shouldn't Temozolomide make the tumors grow faster, if they increase driver mutations? We don't see that.

Now, let's put a face on this:

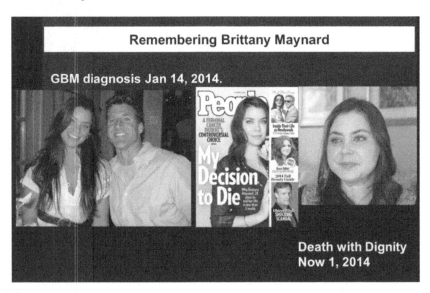

Okay, so this is Brittany Maynard. She was a young California girl, northern California, diagnosed with brain cancer in January 2014. The tumor was a small, a low-grade tumor. And within one month after taking out the low-grade tumor, it morphed into a glioblastoma multiforme.

She was then treated with "standard of care", heavy doses of steroids. And you can see her face on the right there, it looks totally different than when she just got married over here on the left. That's called "moonface", from overdosing steroids.

So she says "I'm out of here!" She's going to go to Oregon, next state up, and die with dignity with her family. She's going to throw the towel in!

And she put an article out, in *People Magazine* about her decision to die! The *People Magazine* article was all about the morality of death with dignity... nothing about the miserable failure of the standard of care that put her in that position in the first place!!

Now, what does it say when your patients kill themselves, rather than continue with your therapy? Not good!

Let's look at another face:

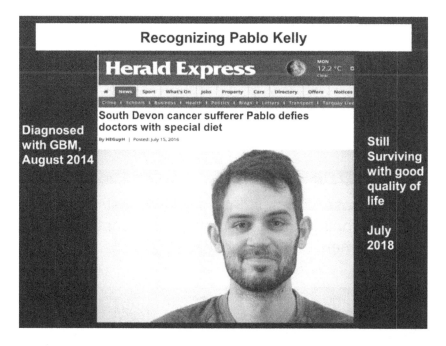

This is Pablo Kelly. Same age as Brittany, about 28. He was diagnosed with glioblastoma in August 2014. He emailed me and says "Can you help me? I don't want to take drugs, I don't want surgery, I don't want radiation. I don't want chemo!"

So, I gave him the kit that I send to most of the cancer patients who contact me. And I said "Hey, you might as well try it, Pablo!" - because he's like "I'm definitely not doing this stuff the doctors tell me!" He's from Devon, England.

He said "Okay, I'll try it your way!" So I gave him the kit. I hadn't heard from him, maybe a year and a half go by. All of a sudden, I get a letter from Pablo: "Oh geez, Pablo! Pablo is still alive!" And he had this big Youtube video, telling everybody how he was going to do keto and all this stuff. But anyway, he says, his now formerly inoperable tumor now has become operable.

So he asked me about it and I said, "Well, if you can shrink it down, get it out Pablo!" So he goes and has the surgery. It was earlier this year, he gets the tumor out. He's had few seizures, but his quality of life is pretty good. His wife just had a baby. He's still alive, he's doing well. Right?

He has a quality of life, he's alive!

So what we did, knowing about all these situations: We built the 'Glucose Ketone Index Calculator' [GKI]. Which helps patients and others get into therapeutic ketosis. So if you want to stop the growth of the tumor, the first step you got to do is:

Get into therapeutic ketosis!

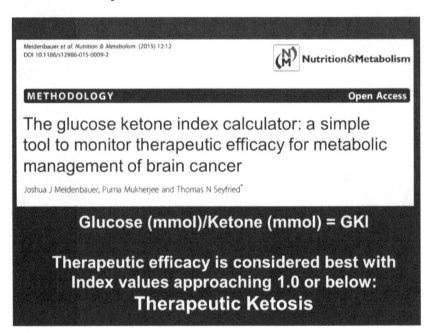

And it's the ratio of glucose millimolar / ketone millimolar, with one of these Precision Extra or Keto-Mojo meters. We're testing all these things against chemistry.

The GKI number helps patients stop the growth of the tumor! So it makes it easier, rather than trying to measure the two fuels together, you get a single value.

We also built some of the greatest preclinical glioma models... the most replicable models to human glioblastoma, spontaneous brain tumors in the mouse. So you know that they're coming from the host

And you can see this mouse, VM-M3 is a glioblastoma. On the left here you can see the tumor:

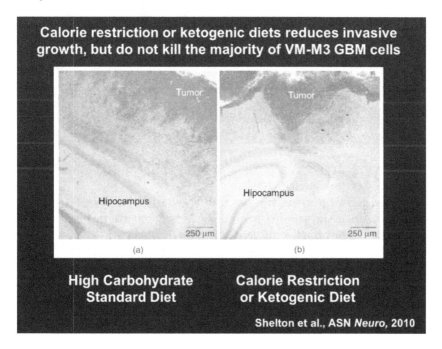

It invades right through the brain using the same mechanisms as you see in humans. On the right is the same tumor in mice, treated with calorie restriction and ketogenic diets. We pound these tumors, hard! Now, we stopped invasion. You can see on the right, there's much less invasive behavior - but we couldn't kill the cells. They're still growing!

I threw everything at these tumors, we were fasting these mice, we were bringing the sugars down, ketones up and the damn tumor cells are still alive! Humans do much better than these mice. I tell you, I don't understand how the human brain can respond so well. Humans are much more responsive to this therapy than the mice. People say "You cure mice all the time!" You don't cure these mice! A mouse that has the same tumor as a human, you get the same problem.

So, I said "These tumors must be using glutamine!" So, we tested the glutamine hypothesis by using 6-Diazo-5-oxo-L-norleucine which is DON. It's been used in the past, it's an old drug, it was used years ago. It worked out for some cancers but not for other cancers, you know. It was just one of those things... some were a little too toxic, some not toxic.

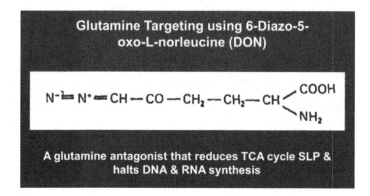

Glutamine Targeting using 6-Diazo-5-oxo-L-norleucine (DON)

$$N^- \equiv N^+ = CH - CO - CH_2 - CH_2 - CH \begin{smallmatrix} COOH \\ NH_2 \end{smallmatrix}$$

A glutamine antagonist that reduces TCA cycle SLP & halts DNA & RNA synthesis

Anyway, what it does is: It stops glutamine metabolism! So we decided to test mice with DON.

We decided to put the tumors into the brain and then let it go for three days until the tumors are raging. Then put them on a fast and then switch them back either to a high carbohydrate [Standard Diet unrestricted calories SD-UR] diet or a ketogenic diet, restricted [KD-R], with or without DON:

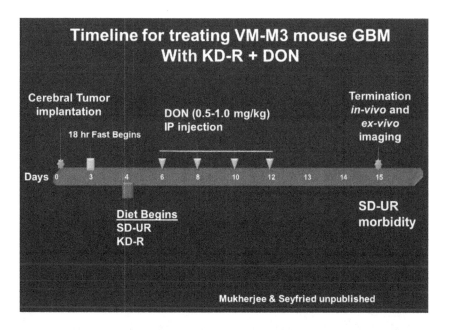

On the top, then, we pulsed DON, pulsed DON at day 6, 8, 10, 12, every other day. We'd give them a little DON while they were on these diets. We stopped the experiments at day 15 because the control mice, they're dying! They're starting to get morbid, because the tumors are growing so fast from all the carbohydrates and everything!

We then compare and contrast the brain tissues and the biochemistry of the tumors at 15 days. And I have to add... we genetically engineered these tumor cells to be bioluminescent so we can see how active the tumor is by putting them into a bioluminescence Xenogen machine. We take the brains out of the mice and we put them in these petri dishes and put some luciferin in there:

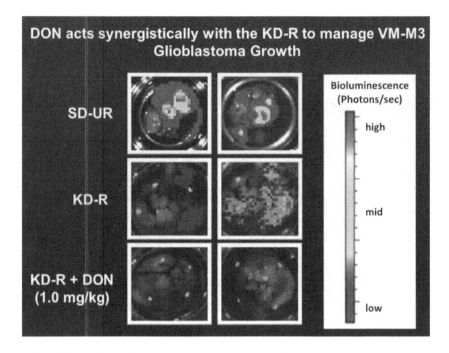

DON acts synergistically with the KD-R to manage VM-M3 Glioblastoma Growth

SD-UR

KD-R

KD-R + DON
(1.0 mg/kg)

Bioluminescence
(Photons/sec)

high

mid

low

The light tells us how many living tumor cells there are in the brains of these mice that are treated under these different conditions. And the mice on the top: You see a lot of bright lights, reds and yellows and all this... They're the ones that didn't get anything but the high carb diet. They're tumors are raging! And we have a lot of different studies to show this.

The ketogenic diet, restricted: You can still see, there's a lot of living tumor cells in the brains of these mice! We did not cure these mice with ketogenic diets. The tumor cells did not invade as much, and I'll show you evidence for that.

But when you add the DON, the glutamine inhibitor, together with the diet we got no light! Right? There was no light! We did this over and over again!

Here's the data of a series of individual mice:

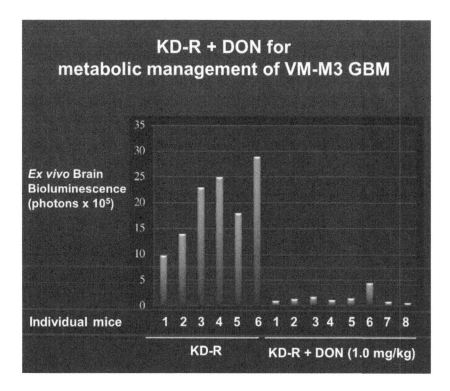

1-6 are the guys that got the diet only [KD-R] and then the other guys, 1-8, got the diet with the DON. And that background light at the +DON group, that's all background except for one mouse there with a little breakthrough light. But by and large, we really eliminated the light and the living cells in these tumors by putting the diet together with the DON!

The DON by itself is okay, but it doesn't get rid of as much light as as putting the DON with the diet. The two together work best. And of course, the gold standard for determining cancer is histology! That's what they, do they take needle biopsies "Oh, you look at the cells you got cancer", right? So you have to do histology to determine what's going on inside the tissue.

And when we did that... here we have the standard diet, the ketogenic diet restricted and the ketogenic diet restricted with the DON:

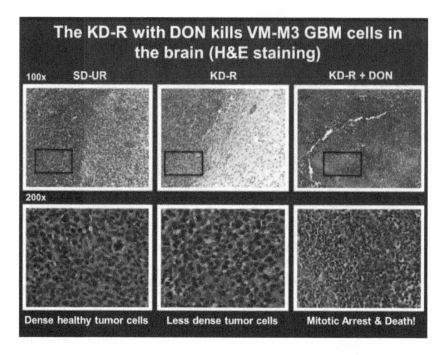

The KD-R with DON kills VM-M3 GBM cells in the brain (H&E staining)

100x SD-UR	KD-R	KD-R + DON
200x		
Dense healthy tumor cells	Less dense tumor cells	Mitotic Arrest & Death!

Low power, high power, is what you're seeing. And if you look at the standardized diet on the left, these cells are piled on top of each other. They can't grow any faster than they're growing! The mitotic figures, the cells are densely packed. And that's what you get when you have a high carbohydrate diet.

The ketogenic diet, the one in the middle, you can see the white part of the brain there: That's the normal part. And KD is blocking the invasion from the dark blue into the white. You can see how much the invasion is over here in the high carb diet. The cells are spaced further apart. So what it's telling us is: The KD is preventing invasion and it's stopping the rate of growth. But they're still growing.

On the far right, you've got the DON and... what we see is: All dead cells! Right? Blasted, the treatment slaughtered these cancer cells! They're all broken, mitotic arrest, they're all dead! This supports the fact that we didn't have any light, the tumor cells are dead!

So based on this we developed the "Press Pulse Therapeutic Strategy" for humans:

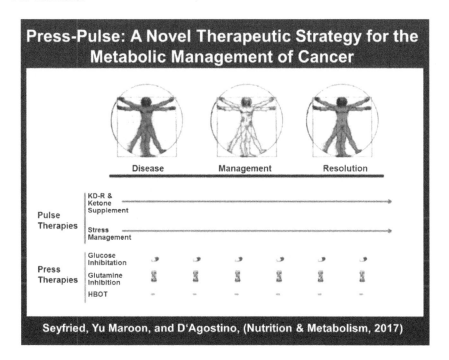

Based on our pre-clinical studies in mice. And I worked together with Dom D'Agostino, Joe Maroon the neurosurgeon. George Yu is an oncologist. And we put this together and, unfortunately I don't have time to tell you where the origin of press-pulse comes.

But basically: We use press therapies, which can include the ketogenic diet, restricted, ketone supplementation - and stress management!

You know... you can't believe that when you have cancer people get stressed out! You have this impending doom,"I'm going to die!" What does that do? It raises your blood sugar - cortisol goes up! You've got to have stress management! So we use exercise, we use music therapy, we use yoga therapy. Whatever works to lower the stress of the individual.

We use the diet as a press: The diet is controlling the availability of sugar to the cancer - and raising ketones, that the tumor cells can't use. Once we get the patient into therapeutic ketosis and lowered stress, we then apply pulses. And we use drugs like 2-Deoxy-D-Glucose, insulin potentiation therapy... we then hit them with glutamine inhibitors, like EGCG (the green tea extract) and chloroquine (the anti-inflammatory). And we would like to get DON, of course, and other drugs.

Then we put them in hyperbaric oxygen chambers [HBOT]. Hyperbaric oxygen will kill tumor cells (just like radiation does) without toxicity! Once you have removed the glucose and glutamine, get the patient into therapeutic ketosis!

So, we can replace the entire standard of care with a logical therapeutic process, that's non-toxic. And we gradually move the patient from the disease state to the so-called "managed state". And eventually, hopefully, to a long-term management and possible resolution using press-pulse metabolic therapy.

Now, how does it work? Okay, so here's a paper that we just published on a patient with glioblastoma from Egypt. We can't do this in the United States!! You can't do this in England, right? You can't do it in a lot of places because of the obligatory standard of care protocol!

So, we had to go to Egypt, where they read our books, they read our stuff and they said "Okay, we're going to try this!" They came to me and told me how they're doing this and they said "Can you help us write it all up?" You know, a lot of physicians can't write papers. But I do this for a living.

I said "We'll get the data, we'll put it all together, just like we do the mice and we'll set up a protocol":

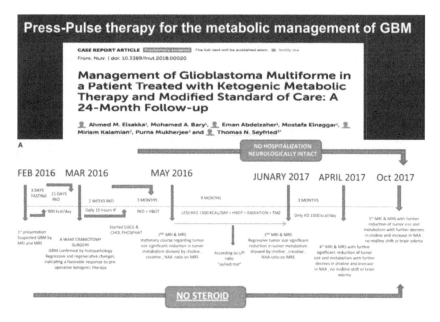

Management of glioblastoma to patients with ketogenic metabolic therapy with modified, modified standard of care. That's what we can't do in this country, so far: IRBs will not allow us to modify the standards of care.

We took this guy, he came in, his whole left side was dragging... he was a metabolic mess, he had pre-diabetes, he had low Vitamin D, had all kinds of other issues... besides, he had a glioblastoma.

So, the first thing Dr. Elsakka did: We gave him a 3 day water only fast and then transitioned the guy to a 900 kilocalorie a day ketogenic diet for 21 days. So he's out over 3 weeks, before we touched him!

Then he did a wake craniotomy. We debulked the tumor! The tumor looks different now! The tumor has a different morphology based on the on the treatment of the diet up front. You're shrinking down those cells!

Then, for another 3 months, we gave him chloroquine, we gave him ECGC, we gave hyperbaric oxygen... Then we were forced into doing standard of care. Because they have to do it! And while he's getting the standard of care - which is radiation and chemo - he's also on hyperbaric oxygen and the diet as well.

And then, for another three months, you can see after that... Now, at 24 months, the guy is doing fine, right? He's a corn farmer, he's back out working in the fields. So now he's out 30 months and he's still doing. I just talked to Dr. Elsakka the other day, I asked "How's the guy doing, the corn farmer?"

"He's doing fine!"

But he had a little radiation edema which pisses us all off some fierce. You don't want to irradiate the human brain, under any conditions! I don't understand that, it kills me! You know, I'm looking at these poor people and I'm saying

"What are you doing?"

"Well, we have to kill the tumor cells!"

"Just take away the glucose and glutamine you get the same effect!"

So here you can see the effect of our treatment:

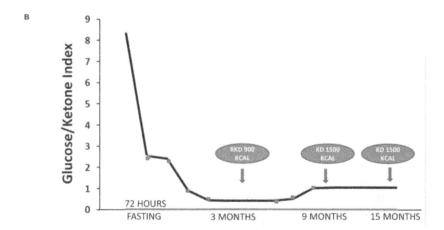

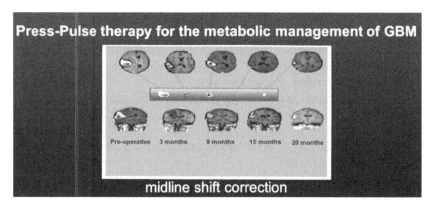

Press-Pulse therapy for the metabolic management of GBM

midline shift correction

Bring the GKI down, glucose ketone index, we got it down really nice, therapeutic ketosis. And on the bottom, look at this: You see the red line on the bottom, see this big tumor there? Okay. Watch as the treatment continues at the very end, you see the red line in the middle is now straight! We corrected the midline shift and the guy's doing fine!

And it's just not brain cancer. This is a patient for a triple negative breast cancer from our colleagues in Turkey, in the Istanbul Clinic. And they're treating all kinds of lung cancer, pancreatic cancer... all stage four, all stage four cancers. This stage four woman comes in with a triple negative breast cancer:

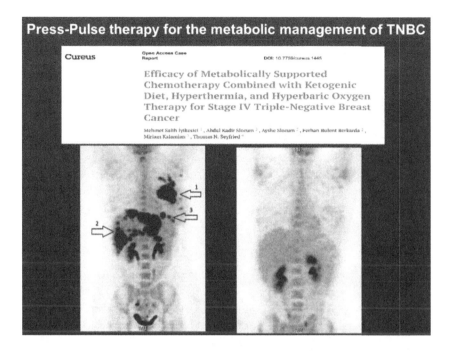

Press-Pulse therapy for the metabolic management of TNBC

Cureus

Open Access Case
Report

DOI: 10.7759/cureus.1445

Efficacy of Metabolically Supported
Chemotherapy Combined with Ketogenic
Diet, Hyperthermia, and Hyperbaric Oxygen
Therapy for Stage IV Triple-Negative Breast
Cancer

Mehmet Salih Iyikesici [1], Abdul Kadir Slocum [2], Ayshe Slocum [2], Ferhan Hulent Berkarda [3], Miriam Kalamian [4], Thomas N. Seyfried [5]

Number one is in the breast, two is in the liver, three is in soft muscle tissue. Again, ketogenic diets, hypothermia, hypobaric oxygen... the lowest dose of chemo possible to remain compliant with the law! I said to Dr. Slocum "What happens if we get rid of the chemo?" "Patient would do better!" But you got to do it! Because you're going to lose your license if you don't. Can you believe this?

Anyway, this patient is doing well! We published in *Cureus Open Access*. We got asked by somebody "How's that patient doing, how's that patient?" Dr. Slocum says the patient is still doing well. Never lost hair, always had a high quality of life, never got sick. And we're seeing this over and over again.

Not in everybody! I don't want to make it look like "Hey, everybody's doing well!" You know, there's a few people who don't make it. They've been beat up so bad by the traditional standards of care, their bodies can't rally. They're so demolished in their ability to heal themselves by the traditional standards of care, they can't heal, they can't rally.

So we have this, GBM and other stage four cancers. I don't consider them as terminal cancers! I don't think they should be considered terminal cancers, okay? Because we're mistreating the patients. We're putting them into risk of death by the very treatments that we're using to try to save them. Makes no sense. You poison and irradiate people to make them healthy? Give me a break!

You've got Brittany Maynard "standard of care" - and then you got Pablo, rejects standard of care. "Oh. They're only one person."

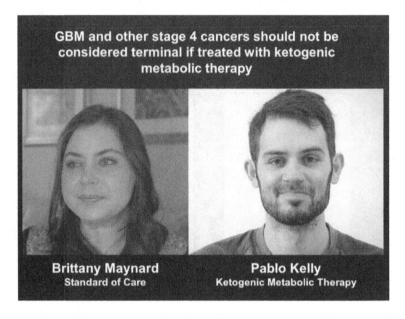

No, there's not one... there's Allison Gannett, there's Andrew Scarborough, there's a whole bunch out there - we just haven't published them yet!

So, Conclusions:

Conclusions

1. Cancer is a type of mitochondrial metabolic disease: It is not a genetic disease!

2. A reliance on substrate level phosphorylation for energy is the metabolic hallmark of all or nearly all cancers

3. The simultaneous restriction of glucose and glutamine can manage GBM and most other cancers.

4. Press-Pulse metabolic therapy is a non toxic, cost effective strategy for the management and possible resolution of all types of cancer!

- Cancer is a type of mitochondrial metabolic disease. It's not a genetic disease!

Okay? This misunderstanding is the greatest tragedy in the history of medicine. Leading to the unnecessary suffering and death of tens of millions of people! By a fundamental misunderstanding of what the nature of the disease is!

- These cells rely on substrate level phosphorylation.

It's the hallmark of what these cells do!

- They're dependent on glucose and glutamine as the prime fuels for GBM and all these other cancers.

They need that fermentable fuel! **Who's targeting the fermentable fuels? Nobody!**

- The Press-Pulse metabolic therapy is non-toxic, cost-effective for the management and possible resolution of all types of cancers

It's a singular disease, all these tumor cells are all fermenters. Doesn't make any difference. It's my opinion and it could be, you know... I don't know if I'll live to see it.... that this strategy will eventually make all of the strategies obsolete. It's just a matter of time.

So I want to thank my collaborators and colleagues from the United States, from Turkey, from Germany, from Venezuela, from Hungary, Greece, France, Egypt, India and China. The Chinese want to now start dovetailing this into their traditional Chinese medicine.

And I especially like to thank our supporters and the funding that we get from them - which is very hard, believe me!

You get massive amounts of money to study cancer, you get very little if you want to try to resolve the disease!

Single Cure Single Cause Foundation [now *The Foundation for Metabolic Cancer Therapies*], CrossFit - thank you very much. Dr. Joe Maroon, team surgeon for the Pittsburgh Steelers, distinguished neurosurgeon at the University of Pittsburgh. George Yu, oncologist. Ellen Davis, Boston College. And in the past the NIH.

Thank you for your attention.

Dr. Thomas Seyfrieds book and paper:

Seyfried, *Cancer as a Metabolic Disease*, 2012 John Wiley Press;

Cancer as a metabolic disease: implications for novel therapeutics

Thomas N. Seyfried,* Roberto E. Flores, Angela M. Poff and Dominic P. D'Agostino - *Carcinogenesis.* 2014 Mar

https://www.ncbi.nlm.nih.gov/pmc/articles/PMC3941741/

Papers cited / mentioned (in chronological order):

1. Hallmarks of cancer: the next generation
Douglas Hanahan, Robert A Weinberg
Cell. 2011 Mar 4
https://pubmed.ncbi.nlm.nih.gov/21376230/

2. A comprehensive catalogue of somatic mutations from a human cancer genome
Erin D. Pleasance, R. Keira Cheetham, Michael R. Stratton
Nature. 463
https://www.nature.com/articles/nature08658

3. Transplantation of pluripotential nuclei from triploid frog tumors
R. G. McKinnell, B. A. Deggins, D. D. Labat
Science. 1969 Jul 25
https://pubmed.ncbi.nlm.nih.gov/5815255/

4. Reprogramming of a melanoma genome by nuclear transplantation
Konrad Hochedlinger, Robert Blelloch, Cameron Brennan et al.,
Genes Dev. 2004 Aug 1
https://pubmed.ncbi.nlm.nih.gov/15289459/

5. On the Origin of Cancer Cells
Otto Warburg
Science. 24 Feb 1956
https://science.sciencemag.org/content/123/3191/309

6. Effects of a ketogenic diet on tumor metabolism and nutritional status in pediatric oncology patients: two case reports
L. C. Nebeling, F. Miraldi, S. B. Shurin, E. Lerner
J Am Coll Nutr. 1995 Apr 14
https://pubmed.ncbi.nlm.nih.gov/7790697/

7. Role of glucose and ketone bodies in the metabolic control of experimental brain cancer.
T. N. Seyfried , T. M. Sanderson, M. M. El-Abbadi, R. McGowan, P. Mukherjee
Br J Cancer. 2003 Oct 6
https://pubmed.ncbi.nlm.nih.gov/14520474/

8. Antiangiogenic and proapoptotic effects of dietary restriction on experimental mouse and human brain tumors

Purna Mukherjee , Laura E. Abate, Thomas N. Seyfried
Clin Cancer Res. 2004 Aug 15
https://pubmed.ncbi.nlm.nih.gov/15328205/

9. Influence of caloric restriction on constitutive expression of NF-κB in an experimental mouse astrocytoma
Tiernan J. Mulrooney, Jeremy Marsh, Ivan Urits, Thomas N. Seyfried, Purna Mukherjee
PLoS One. 2011 Mar 30
https://pubmed.ncbi.nlm.nih.gov/21479220/

10. Dietary restriction reduces angiogenesis and growth in an orthotopic mouse brain tumour model
P. Mukherjee, M. M. El-Abbadi, J. L. Kasperzyk, M. K. Ranes, T. N. Seyfried
Br J Cancer. 2002 May 20
https://pubmed.ncbi.nlm.nih.gov/12085212/

11. Electron microscopy morphology of the mitochondrial network in human cancer
Gabriel Arismendi-Morillo
Int J Biochem Cell Biol. 2009 Oct
https://pubmed.ncbi.nlm.nih.gov/19703662/

12. Does the existing standard of care increase glioblastoma energy metabolism?
Thomas N. Seyfried, Laura M. Shelton, Purna Mukherjee
Lancet Oncol. 2010 Sep 11
https://pubmed.ncbi.nlm.nih.gov/20634134/

13. Effects of radiotherapy with concomitant and adjuvant temozolomide versus radiotherapy alone on survival in glioblastoma in a randomised phase III study: 5-year analysis of the EORTC-NCIC trial
Stupp R et al.,
Lancet Oncol. 2009 May 10
https://pubmed.ncbi.nlm.nih.gov/19269895/

14. The glucose ketone index calculator: a simple tool to monitor therapeutic efficacy for metabolic management of brain cancer
Joshua J. Meidenbauer, Purna Mukherjee, Thomas N. Seyfried
Nutr Metab (Lond). 2015 Mar 11
https://pubmed.ncbi.nlm.nih.gov/25798181/

15. Calorie restriction as an anti-invasive therapy for malignant brain cancer in the VM mouse
Laura M. Shelton, Leanne C. Huysentruyt, Purna Mukherjee, Thomas N. Seyfried
ASN Neuro. 2010 Jul 23
https://pubmed.ncbi.nlm.nih.gov/20664705/

16. Therapeutic benefit of combining calorie-restricted ketogenic diet and glutamine targeting in late-stage experimental glioblastoma
Purna Mukherjee, Thomas N. Seyfried et al.,
Commun Biol. 2019 May 29
https://pubmed.ncbi.nlm.nih.gov/31149644/

17. Management of Glioblastoma Multiforme in a Patient Treated With Ketogenic Metabolic Therapy and Modified Standard of Care: A 24-Month Follow-Up
Ahmed M. A. Elsakka, Thomas N. Seyfried et al.,
Front Nutr. 2018; 5; 20
https://www.ncbi.nlm.nih.gov/pmc/articles/PMC5884883/

Chapter 2

Dr. Dominic D'Agostino on the ketogenic diet and the press-pulse treatment for cancer

(...)

These are the applications for the ketogenic diet and there are many applications that I didn't even put on here:

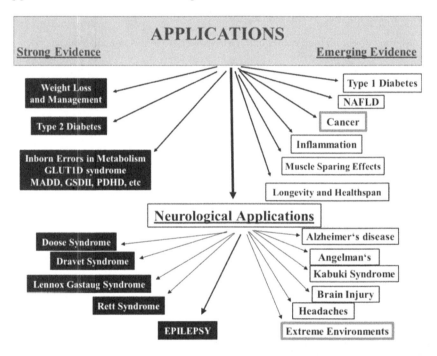

Like the ketogenic diet for acne or polycystic ovary syndrome [PCOS]. Or we study various psychological effects of ketones, too.

So I am just going to focus primarily on cancer... but just look at the emerging applications. And on the left here are things that have really strong evidence in the literature.

Weight loss and weight management, type 2 diabetes I think we can say there's strong evidence for that. Obviously inborn errors of metabolism. The last prior to coming here, I was in Chicago meeting with the doctors who actually give ketones intravenously with all these different neuro-metabolic disorders and they can bring children to life by giving them ketones when they have specific metabolic disorders.

And things like Lennox-Gaustaug syndrome, it's been used for decades for that disorder in epilepsy. I have it in the emerging applications but I think type 1 diabetes, too - there's emerging data from people out there using it. like the group "Typeonegrit" on Facebook.

My PhD student is part of that group and there was a publication that essentially resulted from that group. So there's more data emerging.

And in cancer: 10 years ago, I think there was one or two studies on ClinicalTrials.gov and now I looked this week, there's over 30 clinical trials on using the ketogenic diet in cancer studies. So this is a very emerging field and I think you're gonna see with the current clinical trials, a lot more results from this studies will be hitting PubMed.

It was observations that we made in the cell types that we studied under hyperbaric oxygen therapy and also with supplemental ketones... we observed that ketones decreased proliferation in these cancer cell types that led me down this path:

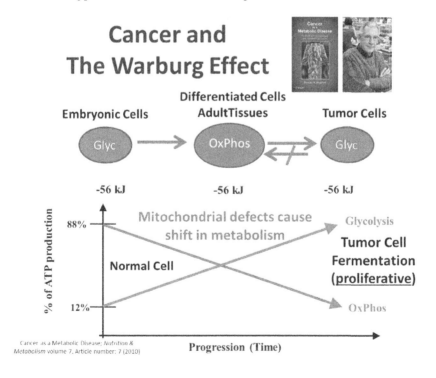

I wasn't supposed to be studying it, I was supposed to be studying oxygen toxicity seizures because we had a contract with the Navy and I was full-time on that contract. But I was obsessed with these observations that we made in cancer cells. And the only thing that really explained the observations that we saw was the Warburg Effect.

Especially the damaged mitochondria and the overproduction of oxygen free radicals as we increased oxygen concentration. And no one had seen that before because no one has a microscope inside a hyperbaric chamber, so these are some novel observations and I needed to explain them. And it connected me with several people including Dr. Tom Seyfried at Boston College.

I read his review shortly after connecting with him, *Cancer as a Metabolic Disease,* which he published in *Nutrition & Metabolism* and then he's got a book by the same name *Cancer as a Metabolic Disease.*

I have published at least seven articles or studies with Tom Seyfried, he explained to me the Warburg Effect which... I had taken cancer biology in college and I had never heard of it before! That cancer metabolism is fundamentally different from metabolism of healthy cells.

Essentially the Warburg Effect in one sentence is damaged mitochondrial respiration and there's compensatory fermentation. So the basic energy processes that allow a cell to maintain its bioenergetic potential would be oxidative phosphorylation. The mitochondria is making about 88 to 90% of the ATP, the energy currency in the cell. In neurons and heart and skeletal muscle, too.

And as a person or the cells are exposed to a number of different agents, they could be
- chemicals
- radiation
- inflammation
- hypoxia
- insulin resistance and
- hyperglycemia

these agents produce a very ripe ripe environment for the mitochondria to be damaged and the mitochondria-DNA to be damaged.

The nucleus has very robust DNA repair mechanisms. The mitochondria does not have as robust DNA repair mechanisms. So if a cell is bombarded with things like radiation or carcinogenic agents, the capacity for the mitochondria to repair itself is not as as high, is not as robust as the the nucleus's ability to repair DNA.

54

So the mitochondria take a big hit. And as mitochondrial function is impaired by progressive damage from environmental agents... viruses, for example, can cause cancer. And the viruses that cause cancer impair mitochondrial function!

So mitochondrial function goes down, cellular ATP levels go down and the nucleus of the cell can sense the bioenergetic potential of the cell, it can sense the ATP levels - and it senses that the cells is in an energetic crisis.

And when it gets to this threshold, I would say... and every cell is different, every person is different. I mean, there's a lot of variables here. But there comes a threshold where progressive damage to mitochondrial function causes a cascade of events to activate a number of genomic pathways that stimulate the cell to increase glycolysis. And various oncogenes are associated with increased glucose metabolism. So a normal cell then transforms and...

We also have to understand that embryonic cells that are proliferating and growing fast also have a glycolytic phenotype. But normal cells that are not proliferating primarily get their energy from mitochondrial oxidative phosphorylation. When the mitochondria are damaged by a number of different agents they will transform. I believe that hyperglycemia, hyperinsulinemia, mitochondrial syndrome is a major driver for this mitochondrial damage.

When the cell transitions from an oxidative phosphorylation energy pathway to a more glycolytic pathway through mitochondrial damage then there's a point of no return. It transitions from a normal cell to a tumor cell. It's debated, but it's not fully understood, if a tumor cell can transition back to a healthy cell. Generally, we don't believe that that can happen, maybe in some cases it can.

But when a normal cell is activated and an oncogenic program and drivers are kicked on, it becomes a tumor cell. And there are a number of factors that can drive the Warburg Effect and actually make that tumor an expanding biomass to a large solid tumor. And drivers of the Warburg Effect can kick on invasiveness and metastasis where those tumor cells get in the circulation and then metastasize. Then it becomes sort of an irreversible process.

So these are the drivers of the Warburg Effect and maybe, I guess Tom Seyfried would say the 'initiators' of the Warburg Effect:

Drivers of the Warburg Effect

- Damaged mitochondria
- Tumor hypoxia
- Elevated Insulin, glucose, lactate
- Increased PI3K/AKT/mTOR
- Elevated ROS and inflammation
- Suppressed anti-tumor immunity

The metabolic theory of cancer posits that it's the initial damage to the mitochondria that's the enabling factor that essentially transitions a normal cell to a cancer cell. There are genes involved, no doubt. But the metabolic control of those genes is likely the root cause.

And now, the geneticists... you know, in years passed it was just linked to genetic alterations. But now we have an appreciation and an understanding (and NIH directed research) to understand how metabolism is directing those gene pathways to actually initiate carcinogenesis and the factors associated with cancer progression, too.

So damaged mitochondria within the theory of metabolic theory of cancer is the initial cause and also a major driver. There's a derangement of tumor metabolism.

Tumor hypoxia: As a tumor expands, as the biomass expands, the core of that tumor becomes hypoxic, damages the mitochondria more, there's more genetic mutations and the inside of the tumor takes on a more aggressive Warburg phenotype. So it's literally fermenting sugar as it grows.

And really people with advanced tumors if they look at the actual tumor, the mitochondria are defficient, they are structurally and biochemically abnormal. And according to Dr. Seyfried and some of the colleagues that I've connected with, when it comes to aggressive tumors they have never found a tumor that has what we would call 'normal' mitochondria!

Damaged mitochondria are really a major driver of cancer. If your mitochondria are healthy they call the shots! Healthy mitochondria will keep a high bioenergetic state of the cell, high ATP levels will enhance the fidelity of the nuclear genome such that DNA repair processes will happen and preserve that genomic stability.

So that's a really important point I think that Tom Seyfried tries to make: The ultimate tumor suppressors are healthy mitochondria. There are different ways: Exercise, CrossFit, ketogenic diet, low carb nutrition, intermittent fasting, periodic caloric restriction - we know that all these things enhance mitochondrial function.

Things like elevated insulin, glucose, lactate, increased PI3K/AKT/mTOR pathway is a major driver for cancer. There are drugs being developed that target this pathway, by Lew Cantley for example, one of our collaborators. Interestingly, these drugs do not work in the context of a normal diet. They need to be used in the context of a diet that suppresses insulin signaling. So the ketogenic diet dramatically enhances the effect of these metabolically targeted drugs, the PI3 kinase inhibitors.

Elevated ROS and inflammation: So reactive oxygen species overproduction kicks on inflammatory pathways which can damage the mitochondria and really stimulate.

Suppressed anti-tumor immunity: As the tumor pumps out lactate and and lowers the pH, that actually changes the micro environment to prevent your body from recognizing that you have a tumor. And the ketogenic diet increases cancer associated immunity. So it helps increase the vigilance of your immune system to recognize cancer and to attack it through a number of mechanisms. And my colleague Adrienne Scheck, formerly at Barrow Neurological Institute, has studied that and published on that.

So for future directions, we had this idea about an approach for a new cancer treatment approach. And Tom Seyfried, my colleague, we've written and co-authored a review on this. Talking about this idea of a press-pulse approach:

Future Directions for Cancer Therapy

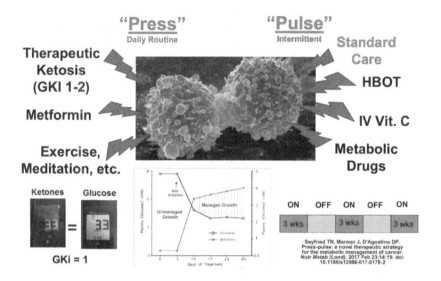

Where a 'press' therapeutic program would be a daily routine of maintaining a high state of therapeutic ketosis.

Dr. Seyfried uses the glucose ketone index [GKi]: If your glucose level is 3 millimolar and your ketone level is 3 millimolar, you would have a glucose ketone index of 1. If your glucose was 4 and your ketones were 2, you would have a glucose ketone index of 2.

We feel that keeping in that 1 to 2 range, if you look at all the animal model studies (especially for seizures), it's extremely therapeutic. It hits all those pathways that I just showed you that target cancer metabolism.

The drug metformin, conceivably, could be used continuously. I think Tom's a little bit resistant against metformin. It may have some side effects.

But exercise, meditation... these things can help you get an ideal glucose-ketone index. Which we know... we talked about the metabolic zone: You bring glucose down to the level of ketones and ketones up.

If you stay within that zone we know experimentally in animal models (and I think the human data will show this and some of it points in that direction) that you are at the very least slowing the tumor, taking the foot off the gas pedal of cancer growth. For the cancers that are responsive to that, that have the Warburg Effect. Or have a 'Warburg phenotype', as we say.

But that sets the stage for other treatment options to be used and our idea is to use them in an on-and-off fashion. Three weeks on, three weeks off.

I am a proponent of standard of care, chemo, radiation and immune therapy. I think for many cancers these can be highly effective and are well tolerated.

I've communicated with enough patients that they get a much better response of these treatments if they're on the ketogenic diet. And they told me the side effects are much less - if they're on the ketogenic diet.

Hyperbaric oxygen therapy [HBOT]: We're just relying on animal model studies now, but... The studies that I showed you from 10 years ago when I was looking at brain tumors, the cells and the mitochondria of the cancer cells were exploding and the normal healthy brain cells were not! I mean, that was very convincing to me that high pressure oxygen was far more toxic to cancer cells than they were to normal healthy cells.

And we published that observation in *Neuroscience* but we really didn't package it as an anti-cancer effect. It was just like an interesting observation.

IV Vitamin C: David Diamond turned me on to this that Vitamin C is a glucose antagonist... Vitamin C at high levels, at millimolar concentration, can be a pro-oxidant! It actually stimulates reactive oxygen species production and oxidative stress.

So it could be used as a pro-oxidant therapy, with or without hyperbaric oxygen therapy. But I think it would work better with hyperbaric oxygen therapy.

And a whole toolbox of metabolic drugs.(...)

––––––––––

Dr. D'Agostinos and Dr. Seyfrieds paper regarding the press-pulse treatment for cancer:

Press-pulse: a novel therapeutic strategy for the metabolic management of cancer
Thomas N. Seyfried, George Yu, Joseph C. Maroon, Dominic P. D'Agostino
Nutr Metab (Lond). 2017 Feb 23

https://pubmed.ncbi.nlm.nih.gov/28250801/

Chapter 3

Pursuing Health #97; Interview with Dr. Thomas Seyfried

Introduction & Host Julie Foucher, MD

Hello there and welcome to *Pursuing Health*. This is definitely the most controversial episode of the podcast that I have brought to you to date, but I'm very excited to share this upcoming conversation with you.

A little bit of background about Dr. Seyfried: Thomas Seyfried, PhD, is a biochemical geneticist, scientist and professor at Boston College. For more than 25 years he's taught and conducted research in the fields of neurochemistry, neurogenetics and cancer.

Through his extensive research Thomas has found evidence that supports the hypothesis that cancer is a metabolic disease - as opposed to the mainstream belief that it's genetic in origin.

He believes that this fundamental misunderstanding has led to failed treatment and prevention strategies thus far. In his groundbreaking text *Cancer as a Metabolic Disease* Thomas explains the metabolic theory of cancer step by step, from the most basic science experiments to clinical studies that support this unconventional view.

Now, although it remains unconventional, this metabolic view of the origins of cancer is now shared by many top scientists around the world and is informing their research on metabolic therapies to prevent and treat cancer, including a ketogenic diet.

I think it's important to share the current state of science with patients and with the general public which is why I was so excited to sit down with Dr. Seyfried for this episode.

Science and our conventional dogmas are constantly being challenged, disproven and changing. As one example: Just look at the paradigm shift that's taking place about fat and heart disease over the past several decades.

I highly encourage anyone with a conventional view of cancer to challenge themselves by reading Dr. Seyfried's text before drawing any conclusions of your own.

So Dr. Seyfried and I sat down at the 2018 CrossFit Health Conference (which was held in Madison, Wisconsin) and there we discussed the metabolic theory of cancer, how he came to this understanding and some of the research he's doing on metabolic therapies. As well as some of the challenges that he and others in this research field are facing today.

I really hope that you enjoy this episode, that it will make you think and that it may challenge some of your current views. It certainly did for me.

Foucher:
Welcome to *Pursuing Health!* I'm very excited to be here with Professor Thomas Seyfried who just gave an incredible talk at our CrossFit Health Conference this week. And so thank you for joining me here on the podcast.

Dr. Seyfried:
Thanks Julie, it's nice to be here.

Foucher:
So I thought that we could start with how you got involved with CrossFit becauseI think that's an interesting story in and of itself. How did you end up here at the CrossFit Health Conference?

Dr. Seyfried:
Well, it was Greg Glassman reading my book with his father. And he apparently felt that the argument that I was making in the book was accurate. Having discussed it with his father, reading almost every page. And then I think his father Jeff had a series of issues with some of the data that I presented in the book and he wrote a long series of questions and concerns.

I brought those to my students, my main associate Purna Mukherjee and we discussed it at length. We formulated a rebuttal to Jeff's questions of sufficient detail to appease his concerns. Because I think Greg has a lot of respect for his father, having had a career in precision measurements... and I think that it became clear that what we were saying was accurate, to the best of everyone's ability to understand the information.

And, therefore, contrasted significantly with the standards of what we think cancer is. And I think that kind of overlaps with Greg's philosophy of, iyou know, challenging systems that perpetuate misinformation and I think the cancer field is one of these.

So he became very excited about this. From what I understand he ran around giving everybody... he bought a whole stack of my books and started giving them out to all these CrossFit people.

Foucher:
He did, he gave me one! First time that I had Greg on the podcast he gave me a copy of your book and he gave me a copy of Travis Christofferson's book. And I think he did that for several other people and really got them to read it!

Dr. Seyfried:

Right! So my affiliation with CrossFit came entirely from Greg and his father Jeff. And it wasn't my reaching out to them, they were reaching out to me. Yeah. And I think that he's been a big proponent of our position, let's put it that way. That's spreading the word to a lot of physicians that, you know, maybe...

You heard the the talks that we had here: Jason Fung's discussion was right on, spot on. They're all on... I mean, there are serious problems here and cancer is one of these. I call it 'the big dog' of medicine. I mean, it's just slaughtering people.

You know, type 2 diabetes is not good, it makes you sick and it gives you all these other things. But it doesn't kill you right out. And you don't have to be poisoned! You don't have to believe that you need to get poisened to get a remission or healing. I mean, the whole thing is upside down, it's just crazy.

Foucher:

It is crazy and I want to talk a lot about your work and some of the things you talked about yesterday. But, just to lay the groundwork and the background for people:

Can you describe what your background was in research and how you ended up coming to these conclusions?

Dr. Seyfried:

Yeah. Well, it's a very long and circuitous route, having been trained in lipid biochemistry and genetics. I got my degree in genetics from the University of Illinois and Illinois State University, as well. I have two degrees in genetics, one from Illinois State University and a PhD from the University of Illinois. These are top programs.

But at that time, we were mostly working with gangliosides, it's a lipid molecule that accumulates in the brains of kids with Tay–Sachs disease. So I was studying that, got my PhD in ganglioside biochemistry, trying to look at animal models that had storage disease.

And then I did postdoc at Yale University and then was on the faculty at Yale, in the Department of Neurology. Their big thing there was epilepsy and they were excited about genetics of epilepsy, so we started mapping genes for epilepsy. Because if you want to stay in that department you better do something with epilepsy. So we did epilepsy and gangliosides, epilepsy and genes, epilepsy and this and that.

But here's something interesting: I wrote a proposal to the University at Yale, back in the mid, late 70s. I think it was like '79 or '78, about using ketogenic diet to work with some of the epileptic models. They replied "Oh, that's passe. Nobody does that anymore..."

Foucher:
What prompted you to do that, just because you were looking at previous research?

Dr. Seyfried:
Yeah! I said "Oh, this might be interesting!" But they said "No, no. It's all crap! Diet is not related..."

Foucher:
Interesting.

Dr. Seyfried:
Only later on, when I was at Boston College, one of my students went out to a meeting in Seattle. There was a meeting on epilepsy, basic mechanisms. And Jim Abrams was there. Jim Abrams is a movie producer for Hollywood. He made the *Airplane* movies and the *Naked Gun* movies. You know, those kinds of things.

And and he was pushing keto because his son Charlie was near death from epilepsy.They started the Charlie Foundation. And early on, Meryl Streep (a friend of Jim Abrams) did this *First Do No Harm* movie. Which was about physicians that were pushing drugs onto this kid with epilepsy which was actually Charlie and how it was harming him and killing him.

Jim then found the ketogenic diet by accident at Johns Hopkins and they started putting Charlie on this diet and he did remarkably well. And today, Jim's son Charlie has graduated from college. He's doing really well! I think he may have been married now.

But anyway, Jim was outraged about the system. One of my students heard all this, came back and told me that they're big on this ketogenic diet again. Not again, but she'd never heard of it. I heard of it, of course I knew what it was. But I said "Yale doesn't think anything about that!"

Anyway, we started... she was so enthused, a student of mine. She was so enthusiastic so I said "Alright, we'll try it." This is at Boston College.

Foucher:
So it shows: Enthusiasm can go a long way when you're a student.

Dr. Seyfried:
Yeah. Well, she was very persuasive, "Let's look at it again". But while I was at Yale, I was also doing a lot of lipid research and we were looking at tumors for gangliosides, anyway. That had changed, as one of the people I was working with noted that gangliosides are abnormal

in tumors. So we made some models of brain cancer while I was at Yale and started looking at gangliosides in the brain tumors.

The work was mostly related to the biochemical abnormalities in the tumors. But at the same time we were studying the genetics of epilepsy. So when I left Yale (I took professorship at Boston College) we started to rebuild the whole program from Yale to Boston College.

And we built the animal models, developing more animal models of brain cancer. But at the same time we started ketogenic diets, mapping genes, and then we morphed into using the ketogenic diet for cancer.

However, it started first with doing calorie restriction. Because Dr. Mukherjee joined me in 1999 and she was a big calorie restriction guy. And we actually...

It was very funny, I think it's in Travis's book, too. Because he asked me how I got into this as well. You know, all of these things were going on, but they were not overlapping.

But in our work on gangliosides there was this drug, NBDNJ, that looked like it was impacting Tay–Sachs disease. And I was studying gangliosides, which is the origin of what these lipid storage diseases are.

So by chance, one of my students, myself or somebody... we decided to take this drug and give it to mice that had brain tumors. Just to see if we could change the pattern of gangliosides in the tumor.

Because we had studied gangliosides in tumors, now we were studying Tay–Sachs disease and gangliosides. And my colleague Frances Platt from Oxford University in England had said "Hey, we got this drug, it's really exciting!"

So I had the drug, they sent it to me. And for whatever reason... because, in those days, we had a free animal cost. Now they cost us a fortune! So we were able to do things that we wouldn't do today anymore. Like "Just try it!", didn't write up a protocol, just do it.

And all of a sudden the damn tumors shrunk! On the animals that were being treated it with a ganglioside synthesis inhibitor drug. So I called the company that was making it. Frances, my colleague, told them "Hey, they found this drug could actually shrink tumors!"

So of course now, the company was very interested! Tay–Sachs disease is an orphan disease. It's out of a hundred thousand people one gets this disease. It's a devastating disease to the kids. I mean, let's be honest. And we're still working on it, by the way.

But, of course the company "Oh wow!" - because cancer is massively bigger than Tay–Sachs disease. So they heard that I had found that this ganglioside drug shrunk tumors. So they asked me "How much money do you need? Just tell me the check and I'll write it out, because we want you to explore this!" So I said "Hm, maybe 200,000 dollars." "Not a problem!" They gave me the $200,000 immediately! It was like the next day the check came in to the University for my research.

So we started then more detailed analysis of the drug. And sure enough, we give the mice to drug and they would eat the food...but we noticed that their body weights were getting smaller, okay? In fact, I hired Purna to help me with this drug work because she had been doing a lot of animal work with calorie restriction and all this stuff.

So she came in and said "The drug has an anti-angiogenic effect!" - which is even more powerful, which is more exciting. It shrinks blood vessels and all this. But we all noticed that the animals that were eating the drug, their body weights were getting lower.

But then somebody said "Well, you got to be really careful about some of these drugs because they induce an indirect calorie restriction!"

So I said "Okay, let's set up a new experiment: We're going to have
- Animals that get no drug - their tumors grow like crazy. (Group 1)
- Animals that get the drug - their tumors are much smaller. (Group 2)
- And a third group: Animals that don't get the drug but restricted food to equal the body weight of the drug group. (Group 3)

And the results of group 2 and 3 came out exactly the same! So the drug had actually no effect on anything other than the fact that it made the mice eat less food! And their body weights shrunk and that was all an indirect calorie restriction effect.

Foucher:
The company probably wasn't too excited about that!

Dr. Seyfried:
Yes, they were quite livid! So they tried to tell me that "Well, when you write it up you got to just focus on the change of the gangliosides in the tumor because that's what's going to be exciting!" Yes, the drug did change gangliosides in the tumor. But that wasn't the therapeutic effect. That wasn't why it was working. It was working because it induced calorie restriction.

And then we went on to show later on, that calorie restriction lowers blood sugar and elevates ketones. Then we fell back on Warburg who found the same thing many years before us.

I said "What's going on here?" It works, because the calorie restriction lowers blood sugar. Warburg said sugars are driving the tumors and they have a defective respiration.

So when we published the paper they said, "Don't put the calorie restriction stuff in there!" and I said that I had to do it. "I'm not gonna lie, this is the main part!" They were upset about it, of course, and they pulled the plug. No more money. Because we actually had found a mechanism that wasn't sexy, basically.

Foucher:
Wasn't gonna make them any money.

Dr. Seyfried:
No, this was not going to make them any money - when you can get the same effect by eating less food, you know! So they dumped us on that.

Foucher:
So you had then found out more about Warburg's work through this?

Dr. Seyfried:
Yeah. Well, at the time I did not know too much. I had heard of him, everybody heard of Warburg. Warburg is just his name, *Warburg*, because he built the apparatus. Like, it's just the *Warburg machine* the *Warburg* this and that. And he had been a major figure. But, you know, as a geneticist and as a lipid biochemist in epilepsy and gangliosides, Warburg's work never really came into our research at all. But when we found out aboutthe glucose stuff...

Linda Nebeling (whose work I referenced) did a paper in 1995: She treated little kids with brain cancer based on Warburg's theory of lowering blood sugar and elevating ketones.

Warburg didn't talk too much about ketones but he certainly talked about blood sugar. So we were seeing the same thing in these mice that were getting the so called 'special drug', that was lowering blood sugar and elevating ketones. And I said "Well, that's just what we use ketogenic diets for: To lower blood sugar and elevate ketones in the kids to stop their seizures."

I said "This drug is doing the same thing and stopping the growth of the tumor!" Warburg said "It's all because the cancer cells have damaged respiration." So we went back and looked at Warburg's hypothesis and theory very carefully and we said "Warburg! This guy's probably right"

Foucher:
And can you explain for people listening who aren't familiar what his theory is and how that differs from our current conventional conception?

Dr. Seyfried:
Well, Warburg made the seminal discovery that all cancer cells produce large amounts of lactic acid. And that's confirmed over and over again, everywhere. And the PET scans, fluorodeoxyglucose-PET scans, light up tumors because they're sucking down so much glucose. But they're also blowing out lactic acid.

And Louis Pasteur in the 1800s made the fundamental discovery that yeast cells are fermenting. They produce a lot of lactic acid. But as soon as oxygen comes in, they stop fermenting and they respire. They don't produce lactic acid anymore, with oxygen. And that's called the Pasteur Effect. And Warburg had mentioned this Pasteur Effect and he argued the cancer cells have a defective Pasteur Effect.

Because even if you put oxygen into the environment, unlike the yeast, the cancer cell continues to make lactic acid even though the oxygen is present. So, clearly, deviating from what Louis Pasteur had said. And Warburg said "Well, how do you explain that? Why would a cancer cell continue to ferment when oxygen is present?" And he put these cancer cells in 100% oxygen and they still made lactic acid, which is incredible!

He came to the major conclusion that their respiration is defective. And the reason why they have to ferment is because they can't respire. He went through elegant experiments, one after another, looking at normal tissues, cancer tissues, all kinds of stuff. And he came to this conclusion that respiration is defective and that's the reason why they ferment.

A lot of people today, even today, don't believe that! They think Warburg was wrong. Only because if Warburg is right almost everybody else is wrong! So they have to defend the status quo by saying Warburg is wrong - with minimal information or misinformation about his theory. That's going on today from some of the top medical schools, arguing that Warburg was wrong.

I wrote the book to prove that Warburg was in fact right! And I went through massive amounts of data, from hundreds of experiments, over decades of research. From electron microscopy, protein chemistry, lipid chemistry, everything.

We have done research in our lab to show that respiratory systems in mouse tumors are defective - no question about it! And that's the reason they ferment, exactly supporting Warburg's theory. And yet, people ignore all this.

It's too devastating to say that this guy, Warburg (who had won the Nobel Prize) was right. He was kind of an arrogant German scientist... he was spared by Hitler because Hitler feared cancer and Warburg was the leading cancer guy in the world. Even though he was part jew. Hitler said "I determine who is jew and not jew!"

Because he decided this guy's could save his life, possibly. If Germany had won the war, cancer probably would have been cured! Of course, everything with Germany after the war was just discredited.

Foucher:
So is that why this theory got kind of pushed aside?

Dr. Seyfried:
It got pushed aside for several reasons. Number one: There had been always a debate about the origin of the lactic acid. Was it really damaged respiration? A lot of experiments that weren't done correctly said it wasn't. Other experiments that were done correctly said it was.

But at the same time Watson and Crick had discovered the structure of DNA. And then they found that there were DNA abnormalities in tumor cells. This was the sexy and hottest thing in science in the 20th century - and everybody ran off chasing genes! And it stayed that way and today we're still suffering from that migration, that lemmings-kind of groupthink migration.

Because the DNA discovery was so profound... we discovered the defects at the molecular origin of the gene. The gene is DNA and the genes control everything and genes are defective, DNA is defective in tumors.

Foucher:
So maybe all this is just about the timing of these discoveries.

Dr. Seyfried:
What happened was: All the biochemists, everybody ran after the genetic defects in cancer and felt that this was the origin of the disease. It even goes back to early 20th century, when Boveri found abnormal chromosomes in cancers and said "Oh, this is probably the origin!"

But even the pathologists said that that was all secondary downstream effects, these chromosomes. And there had been many other papers in the literature saying it's got to be some mitochondrial thing, it can't be genetic. But, you know, everybody was swept away with the DNA and the genes.

And then they started giving Nobel Prizes out to people who were finding oncogenes and tumor suppressor genes and this kind of stuff. Everybody likes to go with the crowd, guys that think they know
68

everything and the whole fields has morphed into this chasing genes thing.

Foucher:
I think you did a great job in your talk this week of illustrating the difference of your approach compared to the prevailing theory to date:

That it's the DNA damage and the nucleus that's driving cancer - versus your metabolic explanation where this is all starting in the mitochondria. And that that's later causing the nuclear damages as a result.

Dr. Seyfried:
That's right. What I did was I rearranged the players in the cancer field and simply showed that all the gene mutations are coming from damage to the respiration. Which produce reactive oxygen species, which are mutagenic. So, basically, the mutations are an effect and not the cause!

So the whole thing, "Where does cancer come from?" becomes much more explainable. It comes from damaged respiration. Exactly as Warburg said. The problem is Warburg didn't know about all of the other ways that cells could get energy without respiration. And we're doing that now.

We're filling in the missing parts of Warburg's central theory, finding the missing link. Which then should resolve all the controversy. Once that happens, then we know exactly where cancer comes from, how it comes and how we can treat it. And that's gonna be a big thing.

The problem is - as we've heard at this meeting - revenue generation seems to be more important than patient health. If we put revenue generation as the prime goal of this and disease management and patient health as a secondary goal, then we're never going to get to the promised land of reducing cancer.

So this is the thing that physicians have to do. They can't be just simply drug pushers for the pharmaceutical industry and I think we heard about that problem here at this meeting. But a lot of physicians allow themselves to become that. Not that they want to become that, but...

Foucher:
...it's just what the system does.

Dr. Seyfried:
It's what the system forces them to do. And once you're in the system... unlike me. I'm not in the system. So I can say what the hell I

want to say because I don't have a medical license to lose. But my friends who are in the system, if they try to do what we think we shoud be doing, they're reprimanded. Or could potentially lose their license for practicing medicine that is not sanctioned by the establishment.

And if you're going to cure cancer, you've got to stop doing the nonsense that the establishment says you should do. Okay? So all this radiation and chemo and all this kind of stuff, you don't need to do a lot of that. You can manage these diseases without toxicity and cost effective.

But, you know, the system is so powerful! It creates... for some physicians, they just have to ignore the truth. You just can't accept the reality that the treatments that you're giving to your patients are actually counterproductive to their health and wellbeing. And you just have to say "I'm doing it because Big Brother told me to do it."

But then there's those physicians that have a moral conscience. They have to be torn immensely within their soul, knowing that what they're actually doing is harmful. And they know that what they're doing is not good. And they also know that there is another way they could treat their patients and they're not allowed to do that! It has to be terribly frustrating for these poor people.

Foucher:
Do you think that there are a lot of physicians who know that? Or do you think that there are a lot of people who just don't see the other solution?

Dr. Seyfried:
I think it's a combination of both. But I think the majority never heard of what we're saying. When you get into the practice of medicine, the practice of your art, you just have so many patients and you have to do so many time consuming things and you're just doing all that. You don't have time to sit down and read the literature to determine whether or not what you're doing is right.

However, it becomes even more difficult because there are many physicians that have the opportunity to do some basic research as part of their internship or residency or whatever the hell they want to call it, it's always confusing to me. But they have that opportunity.

And that's where some of them actually say "Hey, this is not right!" But then when they take it to the higher-ups, those say "Oh, Warburg was wrong!" And if you do that you could potentially lose your grant and you could potentially have a lot of problems. So people don't want to do that.

Foucher:
It's too controversial.

Dr. Seyfried:
Yeah, because you're against the major... The so-called hot thing in cancer today is immunotherapies. You see them advertised on TV in the evening, Keytruda, Opdivo.

Now we even have CAR-T immunotherapies being advertised on TV. Which is an abomination because it hasn't been proven, it kills as many people as it could help! But yet people don't hear that! They only hear what the establishment wants them to hear. And you heard that from Dr. Revins today!

If you have anything that goes against the Big Brother then you will not be heard. It's just that simple. So what is the common person supposed to know? They say "Look at the advances in cancers, we get all these wonderful treatments!" Until they are the ones that have to take the treatment. And then they're asking "How come, it didn't work the way you told me it was? And I had to pay $400,000!"

Foucher:
And you also showed some data at the very beginning of your talk about the increasing death rates with cancer, despite all those efforts.

Dr. Seyfried:
Yeah! And as I said, why nobody knows about this? I mean, this is common knowledge! The American Cancer Society blogs this information every year. But nobody reads it! They all think cancer is... that we're managing cancer real well. But then you look around and see the truth!

And as I said in my book: All you have to do is read the obituary page in any newspaper and you're going to ask yourself "Why all these people dying from cancer?" If we have a solution and it's working why is the obituary page full of people dying from cancer? Makes no sense! It's common sense that it's not working.

And you saw the death statistics: 1,600 people a day dying from cancer? Over 1,600 people - and it's getting worse every year!

Now, if you do metabolic therapy the way we think we should do it, we would drop that death rate by 50% in 10 years!

Which would be enormous, right? Think about it! 50 percent of lives saved that are being currently lost because of a misunderstanding of the nature of the disease. So if you look at... what's pushing the CAR T-Cell therapy, these immunotherapies, is the genes theory of cancer.

So if the gene theory of cancer is wrong (like we showed in our nuclear transfer experiments, I put them all together) then the very therapies that they're telling us will work are not going to work! They do work for a few people, okay? Just by, I don't know, maybe by chance or something. But most people don't respond the way they're supposed to respond. And oftentimes, they can get killed from this. It can kill them!

No physician should ever administer a therapy to a patient where there's a remote chance that this therapy could kill the patient. Or significantly harm them. But they do this!

Foucher:
That's cancer treatment, right?

Dr. Seyfried:
Yeah. But why? Why are they doing this? Because they say "We have to stop the growing cells." We showed that the growing cells need two fuels, glucose and glutamine. If you take them away the growing cells will die. That's so much easier!

Foucher:
Can you talk more about that, about the glutamine and about filling in some of these gaps from Warburg's research? And where you're at in leading into this metabolic treatment?

Dr. Seyfried:
Well, we all know the cancer cells are sucking down glucose. But there are some tumors that don't take in very much glucose and they grow like crazy. So therefore Warburg must be wrong.

But they're fermenting a different molecule, they're not using sugar to do lactic acid fermentation. They're using glutamine to do succinic acid fermentation. This is an amino acid fermentation and it's been well known. A lot of microorganisms do this kind of stuff. But the cancer cell falls back in doing the same thing.

So basically, they're not respiring, can't get energy from respiration. That's why they live in hypoxic environments. They can live without oxygen and this is what Warburg showed. You take the oxygen away, the cancer cells survive. Normal cells die.

Nobody can live without oxygen - but cancer cells can! You can give cancer cells cyanide. Cyanide kills people! Cancer cells are resistant to cyanide!

Foucher:
They'll be fine.

72

Dr. Seyfried:
Yeah, right! So when you put that... cancer cells can live in cyanide, that's what we're talking about! You know, nobody can live without oxygen but cancer cells can because they don't respire, they ferment! And cyanide attacks respiration, it doesn't attack fermentation. So if Warburg is wrong, how come the cancer cell can live in cyonide?

Foucher:
Interesting!

Dr. Seyfried:
People ignore all this. Because it's too difficult to accept the fact that Warburg was right. And then you have to go back and say "Everything that I'm doing is wrong - and I can prove it because we get all these dead people. And if they're not dead, they're seriously damaged from what I did to them."

Now they have to be treated for diabetes management, there are psychiatric problems, hormonal imbalances, gut and digestive issues. You can name it, go on. On and on.

So we have a new branch of medicine called 'cancer survivor' medicine. "Oh wow, we have another whole bunch of people remaining in the system that we can continue to treat with anti-diabetic drugs..." and all the things that we heard here that they're all bullshit.

Anyway, the whole thing... and I agree: I think CrossFit's idea that there's a mess, is understated. It's a big mess!

Foucher:
It is a big mess! I think the more you learn about it, the bigger you realize it is.

Dr. Seyfried:
Yeah.

Foucher:
So for the glutamine, is that something that is consistent across all types of cancer?

Dr. Seyfried:
I think so. I think to one degree or another... not all, because there are some (very few) that don't use any glutamine. It's all glucose dependent. So you take a cancer that's completely glucose dependent, they should be really powerfully impacted by ketogenic diets. A ketogenic diet and lowering blood sugar will demolish these tumors.

But then, the ketogenic diet doesn't work against tumors that are heavily glutamine dependent. So there's where you got to target the glutamine. And if you target the glutamine and the glucose together... we don't think there's any tumor cell that can survive in the absence of these two fuels!

Foucher:
You think those are the only two fuels out there that cancer cells can run on?

Dr. Seyfried:
They can run on other amino acids and small carbs, but there's not enough. If you're going to run a train you got to have a sufficient amount of material. You got to have sufficient sufficient fuel. And if you don't have enough fuel... the cells burn it up real quick and then they run out of fuel. Again, when they run out of fuel, they die!

So you have to have what we call 'logistics': It's the supply of the cancer cell. So there has to be a sufficient supply of the fermentable fuel to keep the beast going. Glucose and glutamine are the only two fuels that are present in massive quantities that would allow this. All the other fuels that could be used could be sucked down in about a day or two.

Foucher:
Okay. There's not enough of them.

Dr. Seyfried:
Yeah, the cancer cell can ferment other amino acids, like aspartate, any of these amino acids. But some of these amino acids, to be fermented, you also have to spend energy to get them into the fermentable state. So to get energy you're spending energy. Glutamine requires no energy expenditure, it's a pure fuel. Just like glucose.

So those two are pure fuels, they require very little other energy. They give you more ATP than they consume. Whereas other amino acid fermentations can take equal amounts for what they yield. And they're not present in sufficient quantity, whereas glutamine is the most abundant amino acid in the body and it can be synthesized from glucose.

So if you take away glucose, you can't synthesize glutamine. If you take away glutamine, you can't drive the tumor. If you take the two of them away, the tumor can't survive. It's just that simple!

Foucher:
And are there certain types of cancers that you know of that are higher in their ability to use glutamine?

Dr. Seyfried:
Yes, there are. There are some cancers that don't show up on PET scan and we asked ourselves what was going on. And they're sucking taking down glutamine! So a lot of the immune cells system cancers are sucking glutamine down big time. Like a lot of the leukemias, myeloids, these kinds of things.

Foucher:
The ketogenic diet probably wouldn't work as well, with those cancers?

Dr. Seyfried:
It works. It works but because it reduces inflammation. It does a lot of other things that provoke... but I think to kill them off big time, you got to target both molecules. So there's a checkmate: You can't move into that spot, you can't move into this spot - you're dead!

So... and who's doing that? No one! We're the only group that actually tried to do this! We did it on a brain cancer patient with good success.

Foucher:
Can you talk about that? About your metabolic therapy and the press-pulse?

Dr. Seyfried:
Yeah. Well, the press-pulse was developed from a concept of paleobiology. People who study the history of the earth knew that in the past there were these massive extinctions of organisms on the planet. And then they would evolve into a new group of organisms.

So they were going back and saying "What was responsible for these mass extinctions of organisms?" And there were two unlikely events that coincided, basically some sort of stress, like a climate change or something like this, that was putting stress on the population.

Some individuals of the population were dying because they couldn't handle the stress, others were adapting to the stress and surviving, but under difficult situations. And then, all of a sudden, like a series of volcanic explosions or a meteorite strike, together with this climate 'press', led to the complete extermination of all organisms.

So you can see where we're going with this: If we develop a therapy that 'presses' the entire body, where cancer cells are under greater stress than the normal cells and then we bring in drugs to 'pulse'... and the pulsing drugs:

We protect the whole body with ketones and put the patients into a good physiological state that kills a lot of tumor cells but won't kill the glutamine ones.

And then we pulse with other drugs that put even greater pressure on both glucose and glutamine, while the body is under the press. This is the strategy. So it's press-pulse.

And what happens is that the patients emerge from the therapy healthier than than when they started! And oftentimes what we see of these patients is: Not only do they have cancer, they have all these other abnormalities! They have vitamin deficiencies, they have diabetes, they have all kinds of other things. All that stuff goes away, along with the tumor!

Foucher:
They get more than they've bargained for!

Dr. Seyfried:
Oh, you get a lot more than you bargained for. It's unbelievable. And they don't have hair loss and bleeding and they don't have vomiting and all this kind of crap. So you can actually destroy the tumor gradually using press-pulse therapeutic strategy. The goal is to gradually degrade the tumor.

As a matter of fact - because glutamine is such a powerful and important metabolite for our body - you can't just take away glutamine and not expect to have other toxic events. So what we do is:

While we're in the process, we'll hit them with the glutamine drug and immediately give them glutamine. Or even give them glutamine, while the drug. Or even before we give the drug!

Foucher:
Ah, interesting.

Dr. Seyfried:
Because our immune system needs the glutamine. So if I kill a whole cartload of tumor cells, our immune system has to come in and pick up the corpses. And if our immune system is paralyzed and can't pick up the corpses... (even though the immune system is not dead, it's just paralyzed from taking the glutamin drugs) but the immune system needs glutamine to do its job!

So you can't just expect... if you kill the cancer cells and nobody picks them up, you get tumorlysis, you get all kinds of other infections! You have to do it strategically. So you want to kill a whole bunch of cells

76

and then you want to bring the same molecule that you just took away. Give it back (because the immune system needs it) they'll come in and pick up all the dead bodies, clear up the system - and then hit the cancer again!

So even though you give them back a little glutamine, you've already cut the tumor population in half. That's good. You've got them under the press so even if they have their glutamine, they're not gonna be able to grow real fast.

So only a few of them will grow but then you're gonna hit the cancer, the glutamin metabolism again and *boom*, another 25-30 percent of them are gone. And then you get maybe another 5% growing back, and hit him again, *boom* another big part is going to die! Eventually, the cancer calles are gone! Right? And it's beautiful!

And each grade that you give, each position, the patients are getting healthier and healthier: They're getting healthier because their tumors are going away - and they're getting healthier because a lot of the other covariables get better!

Foucher:
Inflammation, metabolic diseases in general...

Dr. Seyfried:
Yeah, all these other diseases that they had are also being managed at the same time! So it's a win-win situation for the patient. But not for the traditional medicine! Which is... we should never be poisoning and radiating people to make them healthy in the first place.

And then we put the patients into hyperbaric oxygen chambers which acts as a surrogate for radiation. It kills the tumor cell by oxidative stress. And we heat them up, sometimes. We can heat up tissue which puts more oxidative stress on the tumor cells.

There's so many new ways that we can kill tumor cells. It becomes... you can get giddy thinking about this because you say "Oh, let me try that! Does that work with this? Yeah, it works even better! Wow!"

Foucher:
So many new combinations.

Dr. Seyfried:
Yes! And I think if a physician understood this, their philosophy of treating patients would just be so exciting. It would be almost like a CrossFit competition: You could say to somebody "Do you know how easy I could kill those cancer cells if you do this, on this regimen, instead of that? Now, watch this!"

This is super exciting!

And nobody's doing this because they think it's a genetic disease!

So they build all these absurd things that make people sick and kill them. And it doesn't help the majority of the patients.

Foucher:
It costs a lot of money.

Dr. Seyfried:
Yes, it costs a ton of money, it's just... it's incredible. So I think that the future of cancer is so bright. But at the same time so dim. And that's the tragedy. We just have to get rid of this nonsense. And CrossFit may be one of the ways to do this. It's just amazing to say that, but it's possible. It could happen!

Because if it can withstand the storm that will come... and believe me, you saw how powerful the contrary views are. But I think Greg and the power of the CrossFit community could makea difference. They would need to be part of the spearhead, the tip of the spear to crack this absurdity in cancer that we call "standard of care".

Foucher:
I think we're just starting to see it. This week is just the very tip of the iceberg of what CrossFit is doing. And it's similar to... we've heard Gary Taubes speak as well, about the paradigm shift in fat, the 'calories-in calories-out' theory. And he started writing about that 15 years ago! And now we're finally at a place, where that stuff is going to change.

Foucher:
But the general public still doesn't understand that.

Dr. Seyfried:
Yeah, there's still so many people who don't understand it. But at least the medical community is starting to wrap their heads around it. And, you know, nutrition recommendations are changing.

Dr. Seyfried:
Yes, I agree.

Foucher:
The change is slow. Much slower than we would all like.

Dr. Seyfried:

Yeah and I think we heard today about the nonsense of statin drugs. And don't forget: Not long ago, it's just a couple years ago, there was some guy (can't remember his name) who said that everybody who reaches 50 years of age should start on statin drugs! Whether they have any disease or not!

Foucher:

So can you talk a little bit about your research? I know in your lab you focus mostly on mice, right? Mice models...

Dr. Seyfried:

Yeah

Foucher:

...but I know that you work with physicians all over the world in different groups who are implementing or have implemented your press-pulse therapy in patients.

So can you just talk about where we're at in that stage? And then maybe about some of the challenges to being able to implement this on a larger scale with humans?

Dr. Seyfried:

Well, I think where we have less rigidity... and I'm just saying less, not no. Because everywhere we go, we're locked by this absurdity of the standard of care. And therefore we have to modify it.

We can do modifications easier in some other clinics that we can in in the so-called 'westernized clinics' where you don't have any leeway. It's written in stone and granite and you can't change it. At least, so far, we can't change it.

But when we go to other places, we can modify it. And when we modify it, bringing in metabolic therapy, I think the results are so much more positive and so much more remarkable.

Foucher:

When you're saying using metabolic therapy, do you mean metabolic therapy alone or in conjuction with other therapies?

Dr. Seyfried:

So far we have not been able to use metabolic therapy alone. In any clinic. We've always been yoked by having to use some standard of care. Because everybody has become so brainwashed to think that standard of care or some aspect of standard of care is still good.

In my view it's all bunk! Because the purpose of standard of care is kill tumour cells. And if you can kill tumor cells without toxicity why would you want to use anything that has toxicity associated with it? But they can't accept that, they don't know about it, they don't understand. It's not that complicated!

I mean, if lay people can understand it, more conclusively than the professionals, what does that say? I mean... right?

Foucher:
Professionals often overcomplicate things.

Dr. Seyfried:
Well, even if they're not overcomplicating it, they can't. They're not allowed to. Okay? They're restricted in what they're capable of doing.

And then when people argue "Oh, this metabolic therapy hasn't been proven!" Well, it's been proven at the basic science level. Unquestionably! The basic science says that this is the way to do it! The preclinical systems say this is the way to do it. The only people who are not doing it is in the clinical systems because they say "It hasn't been vetted by a clinical trial!"

Okay. So when you do a clinical trial on a metabolic therapy, it's very very difficult to get anybody to do it. And if they do allow it to be done, it's got to be some stage four terminal cancer when the patient's already been beat to hell by drugs, by radiation and chemo.

And then we're going to take them and then we're going to try to rally all their body, to try recover from all the damage that you've already done to it... oh, and besides: Trying to manage this now outrageously growing cancer that was created by the very standards of care!

So now you're expecting this metabolic therapy to correct everything...

Foucher:
A tall order.

Dr. Seyfried:
... a tall order. But in fact it can be done in some cases. But the bigger issue, as I mentioned: We can't do the critical control group. That's not allowed. It's taboo, but the critical control group would have to be a metabolic therapy *without* standard of care.

What would happen if the metabolic therapy without standard of care is superior to both standard of care and the combination of metabolic therapy with standard of care? Metabolic therapy by itself trumps out chemotherapy, radiation therapy and immunotherapy. Beats them all! Right? What would happen?

Foucher:
Yeah, then we'd have a great problem for our current industry.

Dr. Seyfried:
I know exactly what's going to happen: These people are going to do a hell of a lot better! You saw Pablo Kelly! He's only one of many, you know. They're rejecting standard of care and they're surviving!

Now, you don't go and do nothing. Standard of care is still better than eating big jelly donuts. But if you don't eat the jelly donuts and you do metabolic therapy you're going to trump standard of care. I have no doubt about it, it I've seen it work. It's just unbelievable.

So, we just have to get physicians that understand…

Number one: Understand. And number two: Are allowed to practice what they should be doing. And if you don't understand it and you're not allowed to do it, you're not going to do it.

Foucher:
Right. So it sounds like today most of the experience with this is just in individuals who say "I don't want to do the standard of care and I want to try this instead!" And it can't be part of a traditional research study per se because you're not allowed to forego the standard of care in research.

Dr. Seyfried:
Yeah. But when we do standard of care in brain cancer, we see that everybody who gets radiation dies. Over and over again. Everything you see, people are getting standard of care, 98% of all the people are dead within six years. That's solid data. Nobody's gonna argue with that because it's been repeated thousands and thousands of times.

And you come along and you get a guy who decides not to do this and he lives much longer than you would expect. They still say "Well, we can't consider him at all because he's not part of a clinical trial."

But you still have a few functional brain cells! So if you're the patient, you can say "What the hell? How could that guy survive so long? I want to do what he's doing!" Right? "Maybe it will work! And what about this guy? Did the same thing, he's doing well! And what about that guy over there?"

Still, the establishment is going to say "Well, we can't consider those because they're not part of a clinical trial." "So what? They're alive and they have good quality of life. I want to do what they're doing! I don't give a shit about the clinical trial!" You know. It's just common sense!

And besides cancer: People want to live! I mean, this is not some incidental thing, nobody goes "Well, I'll put it off...", you know. No no. Cancer patients are going to demand "I want to do what those guys are doing so I can stay alive!" And then you go to your physician and you say "Hey, I don't want all that standard of care, cause it could harm me!"

And one of the things we don't know... I haven't seen any statistics on this, yet: Of the people who take standard of care and die, it's not clear how many people are dying from the disease or from the treatments. That has always been a mystery. Because we don't know.

Doctors say "He was treated aggressively... and then he died." Well, how do we know that it was the cancer? Because there are so many radical remissions of cancer in people who don't take standard of care!

And Kelly Turner did this book, *Radical Remissions*. There were a lot of things that were associated with those remissions, but one of the things was radical changes in diet. That was one of the things that was most common in people who had radical cancer remission. A radical change in diet! Oh, does that say something?

Foucher:
Yeah, interesting.

Dr. Seyfried:
Right? But as a physician in the system you're not allowed to consider that. Because it hasn't been vetted. And those double-blind crossovers that are required for standard of care, or to put a new therapy into place, this setup is designed to keep the status quo.

The requirements are designed to only allow another drug to replace a drug that's already there. Not a completely different system. Not a completely different paradigm of treating cancer.

Because there's no way to know if our therapy is the best treatment when those studies can't be done! Our guy's not eating for three days, he's in an hyperbaric chamber, he's eating fat when he does eat.

It's completely impossible to get those studies done without the standard of care stuff! You just have to say based on the hard science, the preclinical studies, the case reports that are published: "We should just do it!"

Foucher:
Let's just do it!

Dr. Seyfried:
Yeah, let's just do it! And have the appropriate control groups. The only group we can't have is the 'know-nothing group'. Okay? We can't just not treat people. So, we have

- the standard of care (which we have massive evidence for)
- metabolic therapy combined with the standard of care. And then we have
- metabolic therapy by itself.

So that kind of a controlled study would solve this problem. That would give us the data that would tell us which treatment is better. Now, who's gonna pay for that?

Foucher:
Right, who's gonna pay for that and also, again, being a vulnerable population, people who are diagnosed with cancer and, like you said, are very desperate to try anything that will work. That poses some challenges as well.

Dr. Seyfried:
Yeah. But when you look at all the things up until now: Nothing has worked!

Foucher:
Yeah.

Dr. Seyfried:
The patients are not told that. They're just told "This is the new drug, we got something new. It could work," you know.

But all the other hundreds of drugs didn't work. Almost nothing that's come out of the genome sequencing has worked. The evidence that the treatment you're going to get is not going to work is overwhelming! Right? Well, we have all this other stuff on metabolic therapy that shows that these people can do really well. Why would you not want to take that?

The turkish group, they only take stage four cancers, so-called "terminal cancers" and keeping these people alive for much, much longer - at a higher quality of life. And with some people it maybe even resolved! You can't know, because it's just been recent, we haven't started this up until recently.

You've got to wait 10, 12 years to know. If the guy is alive and he's doing well and he has no adverse effects from the treatments and he's doing fine, then you get more and more of these people. The ex-patients will get on the web and say "Hey, if you do this, you're gonna survive!"

All of a sudden the patient's gonna come to the physician and say "Thank you, but I want the metabolic therapy."

"We don't do that."

"What the hell! I'm gonna go somewhere where they do it. I'm gonna go to CrossFit, they do it over there!"

Foucher:
That's right. And I know you get emails all the time from people who have a cancer diagnosis. Or maybe there's people listening who just recently had a cancer diagnosis and they are hearing this and they're wondering "Where do I go from here? What should I do?"

Dr. Seyfried:
Well, I send them a kit with information on glucose-ketone index calculators. Because a person... just like Jason Fung was telling, the power is in your hand. If you can get yourself into therapeutic ketosis, you're on the right step. Okay?

Then once you're there, you can think about your next step. But you kind of have the physician to move you to the next step... you can't just put your ass into a hyperbaric oxygen chamber. Well, actually that's not completely true. There are people who are renting them for their homes.

Foucher:
Oh, really?

Dr. Seyfried:
They get in there, they tighten it up and they turn the gas on, or have somebody in the family turn the gas on.

Foucher:
Wow!

Dr. Seyfried:
But you'd like to be in a professional setting to do hyperbaric oxygen. And the problem is that they're not generally part of the treatment.

Here's another bizarre thing: If you get irradiated for cancer treatment and your gut is all damaged and your body is all damaged, the insurance company will pay for you to have hyperbaric oxygen to repair the damage from the radiation therapy. But they will not allow to use hyperbaric oxygen therapy to kill the cancer!

Foucher:
Hm. Not approved yet.

Dr. Seyfried:
Approved for what? Why? What do you ned an approval for, you're gonna take the same therapy?

Foucher:
Right, right.
Except, if you do it before you take the radiation, you don't have to take the radiation!

Foucher:
The irony...

Dr. Seyfried:
I know!
So physicians have to rally. They have to form a physicians organization that stands up to this absurdity. I'm not saying the standard of care is absurd in all cases. Of course, there are some diseases where standard of care is in fact the best, there is no other option.

But in cancer, and in particular type 2 diabetes and these kinds of things... well, I say more 'chronic disease management', this is where metabolic therapies will have the biggest impact.

But you're standing... as I said in my talk, you got the 800-pound gorilla that sits in the room that is basically Big Pharma - and the federal US federal government that's sleeping in bed with the gorilla!

And that is a big obstacle to move. Because the firestorm that comes back, to say... they've called them "merchants of doubt". There's a book *Merchants of Doubt,* the guys who claim that this climate change doesn't exist and all this kind of stuff.... or tobacco doesn't harm you, you know.

They find a study where it's shown that this guy who smoked tobacco never got hurt or whatever... and it creates doubt on the part of the people to say "Well, maybe they're not completely right." So those people will come in and show some guy who does metabolic therapy and doesn't respond - where thousand of others did.

The general public is going to say "Well, maybe most people won't respond to that treatment". And this is going to be a planned undermining of the message.

Because there's organizations that have too much to lose if this now changes.

85

But, you know, as I said: The bottom line is that people want to live, they want to be treated without toxicity. I can tell you now, in cancer: If you get cancer, I don't know if they fear the disease more than the treatment! Because they feel like "I'm gonna have to lose my breasts, my hair's gonna fall out! My face!"

I mean, to people who are interested in their personal appearance this is devastating!

Foucher:
Yeah, and let alone how you feel. You're feeling weak all the time.

Dr. Seyfried:
Yeah, you're sick all the time. Fatigue, nausea. Your hair is falling out, you're gonna get your breasts removed, your colon cut out. I mean, this is like... give me a break!

"I got to be on Imodium for the rest of my life, I got to carry a colostomy bag. I'm gonna lose my arm! My whole life will change!"

Foucher:
Not a good situation.

Dr. Seyfried:
No! It's devastating! Completely devastating! I put a lot of that in my book in the first chapter. About what it means to have cancer and all these different images. You can look at it as a genetic disorder and look at a whole bunch of gene mutations - and nobody gets freaked out looking at a whole bunch of little spots or graphs, right?

But when you see a woman with a mastectomy, no hair and all this kind of stuff then you start to see the real impact of what the hell is going on.

Foucher:
Yeah, and what it does to your family and your financial situation and all of those other things.

Dr. Seyfried:
Yeah, that's terrible. And with the new push on the immunotherapies... it's funny that the ones that work best, the people who respond best are the ones to get the highest fever. This has been shown on a number of occasions.

And William Coley did that many years ago when he gave live bacteria to his cancer patients. They got Staph and Strep and of course, that's going to cause a response you get from sepsis: Your body goes into a massively high fever, 103, 104 maybe even higher. Right on the precipice of death.

But if you can survive the fever your cancer is completely destroyed. And he was able to cure a lot of people with advanced cancer, just by raising the body temperature with a bacterial infection. Then they changed it from live bacteria to killed bacteria and gave it to the patients.

And of course their body responded as if the bacteria were alive and they had the high fever and it worked just as well. But they get rid of that because the 5% of the people had fevers they couldn't control and died.

But it's interesting that the immunotherapies that you give today for $350,000, you'll do best if you get a high fever. And the patients who don't do as well don't get the high fever! So what is this "new treatment" after all? It's a Coley vaccine all over again!

Foucher:
Very interesting, wow!

Dr. Seyfried:
Haha! And Coley didn't charge anything for his vaccine!

Foucher:
Free bacteria.

Dr. Seyfried:
Yeah.

Foucher:
Okay, so maybe we'll start wrapping up, but can you give us just an overview of where this field of research is? The things that you're working on, are there maybe other like-minded researchers or people who are working on this metabolic therapy as well? Where are we at in this country and around the world? Where do we have to go next?

Dr. Seyfried:
Well, I think the biggest thing is:
You got to convince people that this is a metabolic disease. It's a mitochondrial metabolic disease. Okay? So that changes the whole ground, the whole playing field, and how you're going to treat the disease. Because if it's a metabolic disease, why are you irradiating people? They say "Because I got to stop the tumor growth!" But if we can stop it by taking away the fuels then we don't need to do that.

Now, of course you are relabeling what the disease is. And by relabeling and providing the evidence that this is a different disease than what we thought... and that the gene mutations are really red herrings, they're epiphenomena! They're very little related to what goes on.

Well, that's a different difficult pill to swallow. After spending hundreds of millions of dollars on the cancer genome project (you might as well flushed it all down). Just to emphasize still how bad it is:

During Obama's administration they had what they called the "moonshot", 100 million dollars given to cancer research... remember the moonshot? Joe Biden was gonna take charge of this, I don't know if he's still doing it. But the moonshot was to... all in immunotherapies. Right?

So I said to people "Take the money, put it into a rocket capsule and send it to the moon! It's not going to help anybody on this planet!" The whole absurdity is that we keep throwing money at a problem, for a disease that we never had. It's not a genetic disease! So we just perpetuate, the 1,600 people keep going up and up and up because we're treating it as if it were genetic... it's not a genetic disease.

The paradigm change has to be:
1. It's not a genetic disease
2. It's a mitochondrial metabolic disease
3. The treatments that you use can be totally different than the ones we're using right now

And if people want to live...

The other problem is we've separated the cancer into several different tribes: Breast cancer tribe is different from lung cancer tribe, brain cancer, colon cancer, all the different cancers. They all think everybody has a different genetic disease. It's all the same!

Once the tribes get together and become united and march on Washington... just like the Million Man March and the Women March and these kind of marches, we have to get the Cancer March. Believe me, it'll happen real quick, you know. It'll happen real quick.

You got all these politicians that are all bought off by the pharmaceutical industry. They're gonna have to say "Hey, listen, they're gonna burn my house down if I don't do something quick!"

Foucher:
Right. And everyone has someone in their life who's been affected by it.

Dr. Seyfried:

Yeah, Well, I think what that does is: You get an outrage on the part of the survivors. Or the people that even have the disease. There's an outrage, an anger that's unquenchable.

Because if you look at your loved ones who have passed away and suffered as horrificly as they have and then you realize they never needed to do that in the first place and you're sitting there thinking "What the hell happened here?" There has to be some outrage! And the outrage is going to motivate the population to do something!

But if the population is complicit with suffering and being treated for a disease they don't have, then there's nothing anybody could about that. Then we're just saying "Okay, whatever." Just like a bunch of sheep, "We'll just take it, we're gonna just have to toughen up, be poisoned, irradiated." Even though we know we don't have that kind of a disease!

We have an epidemic of cancer all over the world, perpetuated by a misunderstanding of what the nature of the disease is. And it has built an infrastructure of massive financial dominance to keep the status quo on that disease. And the people are just being fed misinformation on television, all this kind of stuff.

So it's a big problem. It's really big and if CrossFit can make a dent in this, my hats off to them.

Foucher:

Well, thank you! I was just gonna say thank you for shedding light on this and for writing your book and for doing the due diligence to bring this information to more people. It's because of that that CrossFit can use their platform to then try to spread it to more people. And help to bring the information out there.

Dr. Seyfried:

I think that CrossFit is morphing into something different than what it might have been at the very beginning. You know, at first it was just keeping people physically fit.

Now it seems to be striking at the very heart of chronic diseases. With a philosophy that goes not only for the diet or for the exercise... but now, it's even branching out into recognizing alternative approaches that might even be better. And therefore, they could be a big voice and hitting far more people than a paper written in *Science* or *Nature* or *Cell*, that only a handful of people on the planet can actually read.

Foucher:
Right! And we're seeing this over and over again, we've talked about it this week, the solutions coming from the bottom-up rather than top-down and from the patients and the people bringing those solutions and taking their health into their own hands. So it's an exciting time.

Dr. Seyfried:
I think it is! There's light at the end of the tunnel!

Foucher:
It definitely is. Alright, I want to finish with three quick questions I ask everyone on the podcast. The first one is: Three things that you do on a regular basis that have the biggest positive impact on your health?

Dr. Seyfried:
Okay. So... I skip breakfast on probably four days a week.

Foucher:
Okay. Usually weekdays, or...?

Dr. Seyfried:
Weekdays, yeah. I do that and then I work out 4 or 5 times a week at the gym.(...)
So if you try to get a fast in, fast as long as you can. If you can get an 18 hour fast, 4 days a week, that's good. And then what I usually do is eat a handful of nuts, like walnuts, almonds, pecans and maybe a cashew or something - and then I don't eat until dinner.
But then I do eat carbs... which I probably shouldn't do. But I tell you, it's just so good!

Foucher:
Yeah, it's so delicious!

Dr. Seyfried:
They're so delicious! You know, rice, I eat rice. I eat potatoes. But we're trying to reduce it more. My wife is more rigid about it than I am. But, I mean, I drink beer. I drink wine, I drink whiskey. It's not like...

Foucher:
You enjoy your life.

Dr. Seyfried:
Yeah! I mean, you try to keep it in moderation as best as you can. But you also have exercise and fasting as part of the routine. So if I were

ever to get cancer, I would be doing a much more aggressive metabolic therapy than I presently do.

There are always some zealots that want to abolish every kind of a risk factor in their life. They won't eat any anything that doesn't produce ketones, you know. Or they insist on exercising all the time. But I'm not that kind of a guy. I don't do that stuff. I go to a bar and drink beer! But not all the time.

Foucher:
I like that approach. You weigh your risks and benefits, you look at where you are at this moment and what makes most sense for you and your lifestyle. And it's true, what's right for you may be very different from what's right for someone else or someone who has cancer.

Dr. Seyfried:
You're right and if I were to have cancer I would be more rigid in maintaining my metabolic management. I'm not doing it now, but... I mean, I do enough. I do it but not to the extent you would do it if you were to try to kill tumor cells.

But yeah, I should be doing it more. I know what to do if I had to do it, let's put it that way.

Foucher:
You're informed.

Dr. Seyfried:
I know where the life preservers are!

Foucher:
There you go! Well, that maybe answers my next question. My next one is: What's one thing that you think would have a big impact on your health but you have a hard time implementing it?

Dr. Seyfried:
Well, I think getting rid of all carbs. Not all but I would say, the starchy carbs. And... it's not easy. You're living in a world of temptations. You go out to dinner with people, they put bread on the table. You can't take the waiter and beat them over the head and say "I don't want the bread!" There's always somebody on the table who wants the bread.

Foucher:
We're constantly surrounded by it. That's hard.

Dr. Seyfried:
Yes, it's hard! You do the best you can. But you know what you have to do if you're informed, at least you have the knowledge base to say "If I do this, I'm going to be better!" Without any information you don't know what to do and put yourself at more risk.

Foucher:
Right. The worst situation is seeing or talking to patients who still have no understanding of what would be a healthy way for them to eat or a way to cure their diabetes if they wanted to. At least if you present that information to people then they can make an informed choice.

Dr. Seyfried:
Absolutely, absolutely.

Foucher:
Last question is: What does a healthy life look like to you ?

Dr. Seyfried:
Well, I can't say what I do is the healthiest. But I can say that it's not the worst. You know, I don't eat pizza every day. In fact, after we heard about the pizza thing at that talk, I said "God damn!" I love pizza, you know! Who doesn't like pizza? (...)
Everybody loves pizza, right? But eating a piece of pizza now puts you at risk for... it takes two weeks to get rid of the damage that a pizza does?

Foucher:
Right, that's what we learned this morning. That changes that whole 'cheat night' mentality a little bit, makes you think about it a little bit more.

Dr. Seyfried:
There's a certain thing... through being happy with your life and not overdoing certain things. But humans are an addictive species. We overdo a lot of things, we exceed in what we're supposed to do.

Foucher:
Especially CrossFit humans. We have a tendency to overdo things.

Dr. Seyfried:
Yes! I mean you guys are nuts with this stuff! But it works, right? But the the so-called 'completely moderate person' is a rare person to be

found, you know. Like my wife, in some ways. She has two wines every night. Never one, never three. It's always two.

Foucher:
She's consistent.

Dr. Seyfried:
Consistent in this moderate behavior. Where I might have three wines or no wine.

Foucher:
Right. The average is still the same.

Dr. Seyfried:
Yeah, but it comes in bursts into rather than... you try to do the best you can. And being aware of this and that's pretty much it. So we'll just keep plowing ahead, find out how long we can survive on the planet.(...)

You know, if you're healthy and engaged, then life is not bad. But if you're depressed and miserable and in pain and... You know, a lot of people commit suicide. They can't handle it. They can't handle life for whatever reason.

A lot of it is metabolic imbalances. Their worldview is just so bleak and so morbid and that shouldn't be! If you're in metabolic homeostasis there is no reason to have these feelings that you need to commit suicide!

That's a big thing, you know. We have a lot of people committing suicide. And you can see post-traumatic stress disorder and all this kind of stuff, that all impacts you. We can understand that, but it also screwed up your metabolism some fierce.

You're on the wrong diet, you're on the wrong lifestyle, your sleep cycle, everything is screwed up. Life is not fun. We all go through tragedies. You have deaths in the family, accidents, you know. You have all kinds of things, job loss, marriage dissolving, you have all these kinds of things.

But if you're metabolically balanced, a lot of times you can handle it. We can do that. It's the people that are completely out of metabolic balance that this becomes too crushing for them and they just can't handle it.

So maintaining the metabolic balance can allow you to survive life.

Foucher:
It's so true.(...)

You don't have to fall so far if you're in peak physical and biochemical condition.

Dr. Seyfried:
Yeah. And it's still hard. I mean, if you have kids and one of your kids gets sick, everything in your life just changes. You get off your schedules and all kinds of things.

But the other thing, too, one last thing is:

To do the kind of research that we do, it's not easy to get funding for this. And we want to thank CrossFit for their support of this work and Travis Christofferson's foundation.

So people who want to make contributions to this kind of work, they can support Travis's foundation. It's called the **Foundation For Metabolic Cancer Therapies.**

It used to be called *Single Cause Single Cure.* Because that's where the support comes from. Because the NIH, they're all locked into the gene theory so most of that money goes to hunt down mutations. Not all of it but a lot of it does.
But in any event that's the way we keep going.

Foucher:
Absolutely! We'll link that up so people can find that link if they're interested in contributing.

Dr. Seyfried:
Yeah, thanks. Thanks a lot.

Dr. Seyfried:
Thank you so much for joining me and thank you for all the work you do!

Foucher:
Thanks Julie, it was really nice. I hope it works and we might help somebody!

Chapter 4

The Origin (and future) of the Ketogenic Diet

In the front yard, on an innocent spring morning in 1993, Hollywood movie producer, Jim Abrahams, rhythmically pushed his son Charlie in a swing. Behind him were the busy noises of his wife Nancy and Charlie's two siblings as they prepared the house for a celebration – it was Charlie's first birthday.

Nobody was prepared for what came next. It happened in a moment. Suddenly Charlie's head slumped to the side, and then out of nowhere his arm shot into the air, as if possessed by some unseen force. Deep down Abrahams knew that something was seriously wrong. A moment before his son was healthy, and now, a fleeting instant later, he was not.

A series of neurological tests proved his instincts were correct. "Your son has epilepsy," the neurologist told him. He then went on to explain that epilepsy, although a single diagnosis, really consists of a wide spectrum of illness; from mild to severe, and within the spectrum the seizures that define the disease are as diverse as a box of crayons. Partial, generalized, and absence seizures comprise the three main groupings.

These are then further parsed into tonic, clonic, tonic-clonic, myoclonic, and atonic seizures. Each category describes a choreographed path of involuntary muscle contractions that spin outward from the neurological chaos unraveling within the brain.

As some time passed, tragically, Charlie's case landed more toward the severe end of the spectrum, and it wasn't just the nature of the seizures, it was the frequency – he was having up to one-hundred seizures a day. It was heartbreaking to watch. Time after time the toddler's brain was taken over while he tried to play. In the middle of stacking a block, or blowing a horn, he would pause, and then slump over, sometimes remaining still, and others with a limb or two shaking uncontrollably. And then it was over, and life would more or less resume where it left off.

It was life lived in intervals. A day was not the seamless continuum most of us take for granted, it was a chopped up into tiny little slices. "It was a fate worse than death," said Abrahams. "The house was filled with tears, all of us, all the time, cried."

Charlie was put on one medication after another – a process that seemed haphazard and experimental. The odds were already stacked against them. If an epileptic child fails the first drug, the chance the next drug will work drops to 10 to 15 percent. Nevertheless, the doses were upped, and the drugs were given in combination; new with old, old with new, but nothing seemed to blunt the attacks. Worse, the Abrahamses watched helplessly as the drugs changed their child in the few good moments he was spared. "You pour the drugs down your child's throat despite the fact there is something inside you that says, 'wait a minute this can't be right'", said Abrahams. "My son was so loaded at times he just lived in his car seat....he was essentially nonfunctional."

The Abrahamses were delicately told by the doctors that Charlie's illness came with additional consequences. The severity and frequency, at this age, would affect the development of his brain – if left unchecked, it would lead to progressive retardation. So it was a race against time. Desperate, the Abrahamses did everything they could. The physician they went to at UCLA, Dr. Donald Shields, was a nationally recognized expert in children's epilepsy. They didn't stop there. They sought a second, third, fourth, and fifth opinion. But nothing new was offered, each doctors opinion was just a reiteration of the last: stick with the drugs. But the drugs simply weren't working.

The doctors didn't seem to share the Abrahamses sense of urgency. Every day was important; Charlie was slowly falling into an abyss. The doctors finally capitulated, and they turned to the option held in reserve: surgery. But the glimmer of hope surgery held vanished once Charlie recovered and the relentless assault of seizures continued. With nowhere left to turn, at the end of the road, the Abrahamses turned to a faith healer. Still nothing.

For the Abrahamses, if any sort of resignation creeped in, it only served to stoke a fire. There is no greater instinctual surge than of protective parents. "After thousands of epileptic seizures, an incredible number of drugs, dozens of blood draws, eight hospitalizations, a mountain of EEG's, MRI's, CT scans and PET scans, one fruitless brain surgery, five pediatric neurologists in three cities, two homeopaths, one faith healer, and countless prayers, the seizures continued unchecked.." But giving up was never an option.

And so Jim Abrahams began his own research. He began combing through books and attending medical lectures. It was an education rolled up in a frantic mission. Then one day, on the bottom shelve at the medical library, he picked up a book published that year by Dr. John Freeman, titled *Seizures and Epilepsy in Childhood: A Guide for Parents*. The book was written for parents to help them cope. But buried deep inside were three pages on a dietary protocol used to treat epilepsy. Dr. Freeman had tried to write a book focused solely on the diet but was unable to find a publisher – so he snuck them into this book almost as an afterthought.

Within the few pages was the remarkable claim that the diet was able to help at least half of those who maintained it. The first impulse that ran through Abrahams mind was bewilderment. If it had *any* legitimacy, why hadn't one of the five doctors mentioned this treatment option by now? "I couldn't make the leap between all these doctors saying one thing and this other guy saying something else," he later confessed. Confused and desperate, he had what he felt were only two options left: the strange diet, and an herbalist someone had told him about working out of a strip mall in Houston Texas.

At the next appointment, when he asked Dr. Shields which one he should pursue, Shields said, "Flip a coin, neither will probably work." And so he did just that, he and his wife Nancy literally flipped a coin: heads the herbalist, tails the strange diet. It landed on heads. The family traveled to Houston and met the herbalist. They took his advice, bought a grocery bag full of herbs, and returned home. After a few weeks of mixing herbal teas it became apparent the strange smelling concoctions were having no effect on Charlie's seizures.

This was the end of the line. The best doctors in the world, the best drugs in the world, surgery, homeopaths, faith healers, herbalists, everything had failed Charlie. Charlie and his family were backed into a corner. There was only one option left. So, with only a thread of hope; desperate, deflated, and exhausted, the Abrahamses boarded a plane to Baltimore Maryland to see John Freeman about the peculiar and obscure treatment called *the ketogenic diet.*

Oddly enough, as they flew to the east coast, at some point in the upper Midwest, perhaps over the Ohio Valley, if the Abrahamses could have peered eighty years into the past, they would have looked down and seen a train heading in the opposite direction to Battle Creek Michigan. On board were their exact counterparts: a desperate family with their epileptic son, at the end of their rope, traveling to the only option left to them – a long shot.

Mark Twain said "history doesn't repeat itself, but it does rhyme." And the stories of these families rhymed in every sentence and verse. But in a larger context, each story, astonishing in its own right, serve only as bookmarks: it is what happened in the interim, the eighty years that lie in-between, which reveals volumes. Critically, it is a vitally important lesson of the infallibility and undulating path of medical science, and a stark reminder that valuable knowledge, even in the modern era, can be lost.

––––––––––

The story of both families converge on a single man: Bernard Macfadden. Although almost entirely forgotten today, in the early 1900's almost everyone knew his name. Macfadden was a bona fide American icon. His rise to fame was also uniquely American, he started with nothing. In fact, less than nothing; he was cast into the world with the odds decidedly stacked against him. His early years were filled with pain and abandonment. His father beat him and his family before drinking himself to death when Macfadden was five years old.

When Macfadden was seven, his mother sent him away to the cheapest boarding school she could find because she was dying from late-stage tuberculosis and was unable to care for him any longer. Macfadden then escaped what he called the "starvation school" and fell into a series of indentured servitudes for distant relatives and farmers, working one-hundred hour weeks and paid only in room and board.

But like all American icons Macfadden fought back, scratching and clawing for a better place in the world. When he was fifteen he accidently wandered into a newly established gymnasium in St. Louis. One look past the threshold was all it took. Inside men were grunting and sweating while they hoisting dumbbells and preformed calisthenics, posters of musclemen plastered the walls. As he stared open-mouthed and wide-eyed Macfadden was at the same time enthralled and infected. Right there he swore an oath: "I'm going to look like them, I'm going to be like them."

Over time, Macfadden parlayed his sworn oath into an empire. Recognizing an opportunity, he started a magazine called *Physical Culture*. What started as a modest enterprise soon rocketed skyward with dazzling growth. It was a fresh, new message for Americans. Within the pages he proselytized health, vitality, and uninhibited enjoyment of the human body. He advocated exercise, healthy eating, and avoidance of tobacco, too much alcohol, and white bread (a substance Macfadden called the "staff of death").

He encouraged nude sunbathing, walking barefoot, and warned of the evils of prudishness – the body, claimed Macfadden, was for unrestrained enjoyment. For the first time Americans were told sex was good, and was nothing to be ashamed of. His magazines were provocative (the first to use scantily clad models); engaging, and told American's there was a new and better way to live. He had tapped into a new niche, he had become America's first health guru, forging a new culture and selling a lifestyle. He was the driving force behind the rise of body-building. He hand-picked an unknown Brooklyn model named Charles Atlas and gave him the title "World's Most Perfect Man", and then was the architect behind a career path that led to Atlas's fame and fortune.

American's appetite for Macfadden's new lifestyle was insatiable. Half way through the year 1900, Macfadden was selling 110,000 copies of *Physical Culture* per month. His rapid success came with a new cockiness. The wildly popular magazine, claimed Macfadden, not only blazed the path to health and vitality, now, it was revealing his secrets to curing disease – *any disease*. His belief was sincere, and consisted of a prescriptive life style that he claimed would bring anyone back from the throes of illness.

The prescription consisted of the principles he had been proselytizing for most of his life: exercise, sunlight, avoidance of alcohol, tobacco, and diet. But the most important piece, the one imperative ingredient to pull people from the ghostly realm of the sick back into vitality, was something Macfadden felt held almost magical healing properties: *fasting.*

Macfadden's belief in fasting, while maybe largely forgotten, certainly wasn't new. Its restorative powers go far back into antiquity. The Greek physician, Hippocrates, made reference to the healing properties of fasting, "Everyone has a doctor in him; we just have to help him in his work. The natural healing force within each one of us is the greatest force in getting well. ...to eat when you are sick, is to feed your sickness." Incredibly, the virtues of fasting, or overconsumption in general, went even further back, all the way to 3800BC. An inscription found in an Egyptian pyramid read: "Humans live on one-quarter of what they eat; on the other three-quarters lives their doctor." (A glib quote that could easily describe the relationship between food and medicine today). Other famous people have touted fasting throughout history, including Ben Franklin, "The best of all medicines is resting and fasting." Mark Twain wrote, "A little starvation can really do more for the average sick man than can the best medicines and the best doctors."

Macfadden embraced the time honored practice that had strangely bounced in and out of favor through thousands of years of history. Perhaps the counterintuitive nature of sick people not eating served to pull it back into obscurity time and time again. Rarely would a grandmother, parent, or a physician in their right mind suggest that a sick person should stop eating – it goes against every fiber of instinct.

However Macfadden stumbled onto the salubrious practice of fasting, his faith in its powers were reinforced by personal observation and trial. While working on a farm, he had noticed that whenever an animal became ill it stopped eating. Years later, one spring he felt the early symptoms of pneumonia stirring in his chest. He remembered the lesson of the farm animals and cut back to a couple pieces of fruit per day. He noticed by the second day his chest had begun to clear and by the fourth day the symptoms had all but vanished.

Macfadden's sideways entry into medicine ultimately culminated in the creation of a sanatorium in 1907 – a massive mansion equipped with swimming pools, gyms, Russian and Turkish baths, and relaxation areas. The Bernarr Macfadden Sanatorium (he had changed his name from Bernard to Bernarr because it sounded like the roar of a lion) was located in Battle Creek Michigan, a small town turned overnight into a beacon for the sick. Directly across the street stood the famous Battle Creek Sanitarium, started by John Harvey Kellogg (his brother capitalized on the health trend and started the Kellogg cereal company).

Three hundred thousand health seekers visited the Battle Creek Sanitarium during its 65 years of operation. Every day the train dropped off a fresh crop complaining of a variety of ailments — a portion of which now headed to Macfadden's new sanatorium with the hope of getting well. Most of those that showed up on Macfadden's doorstep had vague symptoms like headaches, weight loss, digestive problems, and it was really no surprise, the typical diet of a century ago consisted mostly of salt pork, bread, and potatoes. The first vitamin would not be discovered until 1912 and American's were entirely unaware how deficient their diets truly were. Also, the workforce had begun the transition to desk jobs. The combination of a terrible diet and inactivity left many Americans in a sorry state – they turned to Macfadden to help.

At the sanatorium Macfadden hired an osteopath doctor named Hugh Conklin as an assistant. He prescribed to the same belief system as Macfadden. They both believed that medicine, the way it was practiced, was largely fraudulent. Together they called out the medical establishment: *we will take those you have given up on and cure them.* This was fine for the mostly vague and un-diagnosable masses that showed up. After a period of stress free fasting, hydrotherapy, and light exercise in and around the beautiful mansion they did feel better.

Of course, some of the more conservative doctors pushed back, claiming Macfadden and his hand-picked doctors were the worst kind of quacks: "the kind that preyed on those that were healthy but thought they were sick." But Macfadden had star power on his side. Of his more famous clients, Upton Sinclair, defended him vigorously, even publishing a book *titled The Fasting Cure*, dedicated to his good friend B.M.

Occasionally patients with very tangible illnesses, like epilepsy, showed up on Macfadden's doorstep. For the detractors of McFadden, this, they thought, would surely be where he would fail. Epileptic patients, in particular, came with a built-in yardstick. The therapies prescribed would face a true test because of one simple fact: the number of seizures could be counted before and after treatment, thus determining if treatment was effective or not.

It's not clear if Conklin or Macfadden knew the history of epilepsy. If they did, they would have known there was a scattering of evidence backing the idea fasting would work for epilepsy. In the fifth century BC, Hippocrates reported on a man who had been seized by convulsions. A fast was prescribed and the cure worked, freeing the individual of seizures. In a quotation from the King James Version of the Bible, Mark tells the story of Jesus curing an epileptic boy where his disciples had failed. When they asked him why, Jesus said, "this kind can come out by nothing but prayer and fasting."

And so Conklin began to count. He recorded the number of seizures before and after treatment. When the numbers were tallied the result was shocking and undeniable: *fasting worked for epileptic patients.* Once they stopped eating an invisible metabolic levy was raised around the brain. The neurological storms that once pounded the shores were abruptly dispelled. For some reason, however, Conklin felt no immediate compulsion to publish his data. But it didn't matter. Nature abhors a vacuum – the medical establishment had no good solutions – and so word of the "drugless healer" in Battle Creek, Michigan claiming to have an effective treatment for epilepsy, gradually began filtering into the public at large.

As rumors of Conklin's "water diet" rippled outward from the center of the country, doctors continued to treat epilepsy with the few drugs they had. The most commonly prescribed drug was potassium bromide. In the mid 1800's it was thought epilepsy was caused by excessive sexual indulgence and particularly masturbation. In 1857, a British doctor, Charles Lockhart, read a report claiming people had become temporarily impotent after taking potassium bromide. By his own reckoning, Lockhart made the connection: maybe the drug would assuage the sexual gluttony of epileptics, and as a result, stop their seizures? The drug worked in spite of Lockhart's faulty logic.

A decade later doctors began questioning the link between excessive sexuality and epilepsy. More likely, they reasoned, Bromide was acting directly on the brain rather than through the indirect suppression of sexual desire. Bromide is a powerful sedative, and researchers made the irresistible connection between the nervous eruption of a seizure and the drugs ability to slow nervous impulses – like pouring water on a fire. In 1872 one researcher wrote, "The object of medical treatment for epilepsy is to control the over-readyness of nervous action. For this purpose sedatives have been employed with success." The connection was powerfully seductive, and would guide the search for new anti-seizure medications for the foreseeable future. The search for new epilepsy drugs was now synonymous to finding drugs that were sedative – the two qualities were thought to be inseparable.

The next breakthrough happened on a fall day in 1912. It happened because a young medical student named Alfred Hauptman was sleep deprived. The young German, resident-psychiatrist, lived over the epileptic ward while he was in medical training. Below him, seizures tormented his patients throughout the night. He could hear them thrash and convulse, sometimes even the thud of one of them falling out of bed. The unremitting sounds forbade sleep. As he tossed and turned he realized he had to try something. A new sleeping pill called Luminal had just hit the pharmacy a year earlier.

During his medical training he learned potassium bromide worked as an anti-seizure medication precisely because it was a sedative. It wasn't unreasonable to think that Luminal might work through the same mechanism. In the very least, he thought, maybe both he and his patients could get a good night's sleep. And so the next evening, right before bedtime, he gave each of his patients a dose of the new drug. To his delight, Hauptmann slept soundly that night, as did his patients. He would have left it at that, a simple remedy for a good night sleep, but he noticed something remarkable: his patient's reprieve from seizures extended into the next day – *they didn't have any*.

Hauptmann made the connection hovering before him: perhaps this drug, chemically known as phenobarbital, could be a new medication for epilepsy. Once he published his observation phenobarbital began to be prescribed and slowly built momentum, eventually overtaking potassium bromide's position as the first line treatment for epilepsy. Although better at preventing seizures than potassium bromide, for patients, Luminal was still a compromise – fewer seizures was swapped for a life lived in a fog – a hazy, blunted state of existence. Doctor's assumed it was a zero sum game – fewer seizures came at the expense of sedation. It was accepted this was just the way it had to be.

Charles Howland's Question

In 1921, H. Rawle Geyelin, a prominent endocrinologist at New York Presbyterian Hospital, took the podium at the annual American Medical Association convention. Rather than the typical, dry run through mountains of graphs and charts, Geyelin chose to tell a story. He spoke of a young cousin who had epilepsy. Over four years he watched as his cousin tried every treatment recommended by several neurologists, including the boy's uncle who was a professor of pediatrics at Johns Hopkins. The family watched helpless as every treatment failed, including bromides and the newer drug phenobarbital (Luminal). The desperate family took what they saw as the only option left: a train ride to Battle Creek Michigan to see Macfadden and Conklin.

By now Conklin had treated an untold number of patients, probably numbering in the hundreds. Geyelin explained how the young cousin fasted under the supervision of Conklin for three or four weeks. Remarkably, the seizures stopped after the second day, and the remission proved remarkably durable – his cousin remained seizure free for over two years after completion of the treatment. For Geyelin, it was impossible to ignore the result. First, because of the intimate family connection, and second because he knew his cousin had failed every other treatment, the best those in the audience – the doctors sitting before him – had to offer. So Geyelin looked closer. He carefully followed two other patients that traveled to Battle Creek to see Dr. Conklin. The patients, Geyelin confirmed, at least for the time being, were cured – they remained free of seizures after returning home.

Geyelin then took the next logical step. He saw if he could replicate Conklin's results by fasting his own patients. Now, in front of the hushed audience, he presented the results. After fasting 30 patients for 20 days in his clinic: 87% of the patients became seizure free. The results evoked gasps from the audience. The rumors of the drugless Midwestern healer that publicly announce his disdain for conventional medicine were now staring them in the face. It was no longer a rumor; Geyelin had cast it into documented fact.

For the doctors in the auditorium, the treatment of epilepsy remained as frustrating of an enterprise as it always had. "Surely patients with no other disease have grasped at so many therapeutic straws," wrote one doctor. Epilepsy comes from Ancient Greece meaning "to seize, posses, or afflict".

The Greeks also called epilepsy the sacred disease, and as civilizations before them, they thought it was a form of spiritual possession. Consequently, for century's, victims were treated with one pointless ritual after the next. In the fifth century B.C. Hippocrates boldly challenged the assumption epilepsy was divine in origin declaring it was a medically treatable problem emanating from the brain. Hippocrates' declaration would change the course of the disease forever, thrusting it into the empirical arena of real medicine.

But the transition would not be smooth. His declaration started what would be a series of clumsy, barbaric, and sometimes bizarre attempts to treat the disease. The eccentric and unrelated treatments were a reflection of the fact epilepsy was of mysterious and unknown origin. Doctor's attempts to mute epileptic fits were patchwork of trial and error: bloodletting, trephining of the skull (boring a hole in the skull to release the disease), removal of the ovaries and adrenal glands, countless drugs, herbs, and tinctures.

When the Roman physician Celsus witnessed epileptics drinking blood from the wounds of dying gladiators he wrote: "What a miserable disease that makes tolerable such a miserable remedy." And in 1921, as Geyelin gave his presentation, little had changed. "Many Modern 'cures' are not less miserable" wrote a respected neurologist, comparing the state of treatment in the 1920's to those of the past. Doctors still had little to offer the victims of epilepsy; and that a nonconventional osteopath had discovered what might be the best treatment available was met with a degree of skepticism, frustration, and embarrassment.

The father of Geyelin's young cousin, Charles Howland, was a wealthy New York corporate attorney. Shocked that the cure to his son's epilepsy lie so far outside the medical establishment, Howland became obsessed with a single question: *why did fasting cure his son of epilepsy?* Conklin already thought he knew the answer. He claimed epilepsy emanated from the intestines. He speculated that toxins were secreted from the lymph nodes surrounding the small intestine then stored in the lymph system, and from time to time, discharged into the bloodstream, causing seizures. Simply not eating allowed the toxins to be cleared.

Conklin had no evidence to back his claim; his reasoning was nothing more than a wild guess, probably pushed along by Macfadden. Along with many doctors, Charles Howland wasn't satisfied with Conklin's contrived explanation. Instinctually, Howland felt there was more to it. He desperately wanted to know – he wanted an answer backed by actual evidence. In hope of finding an answer, he wrote a check to his brother, a professor of Pediatrics at Johns Hopkins, for five-thousand dollars.

Five thousand dollars went a long way in the early 1900's and Dr. Howland used the money to set up a state of the art laboratory at Johns Hopkins dedicated to the new mission. As with his brother, the question quickly became a particular obsession. The answer, reasoned Howland, was sure to lie within some shift in the epileptic's metabolism. To find the answer would be an exercise in comparison. What did the metabolism of the epileptic look like before and after fasting, and could the relevant factor be isolated from the noise? Far too steep a task for any individual, he turned to Dr. James Gamble, an unusually precise and methodical clinical chemist.

The canvas for Gamble's search consisted of four fasting epileptic children. He carefully monitored every known biochemical variable as they transitioned into the fasting state. He collected and exhaustively analyzed their urine and blood with painstaking detail – from water loss, to electrolytes balance, acid/base balance, and the curious mention of the strange occurrence of two ketones, *beta hydroxybutyrate and acetoacetate*, in the fasting patient's plasma and urine. To Gamble, the compounds were a mystery. He speculated that they were meaningless; the byproduct of the "incomplete oxidation of fats" – nothing more than a useless exhaust expelled as the patients began to burn fat.

In the end, despite an extensive search, the report held no definitive answer, the biochemical shift that reduced seizures in fasting epileptics, for the time being, remained a mystery. As Howland's team continued its frenzied search, about a thousand miles west, in Chicago, the seeds were being planted to offer up a different explanation.

Food Becomes Medicine

Rowland Woodyatt and Evarts Graham, both medical doctors in Chicago, were having an argument over lunch. The waiter was already tense. Their voices were elevated and, worse, they had scribbled arcane symbols all over the table cloth, it was most likely ruined. The argument had drifted away from the scribblings into something more personal. "Your perfectionism is holding you back, can't you see that," said Graham, clearly frustrated. "Did you know it took Lorenzo Ghiberti twenty years just to sculpt the bronze doors of the baptistery of San Giovanni. Perfection doesn't care how long something takes," retorted Woodyatt, in a measured voice. Woodyatt was a perfectionist, in every sense of the word, and Graham was not the first to notice.

He could agonize over the wording of a single sentence, sometimes for an entire day. Graham found this absurd, a waste of time and talent. But for the study of human metabolism, Woodyatt's peculiar personality trait was perhaps his greatest strength. He was intensely passionate about the details. He could zero in, focus with singular purpose, and not allow himself to be railroaded by the incredibly complex maze of metabolic pathways where others quickly became overwhelmed.

In the summer of 1921, Woodyatt's passion for metabolism culminated in an article titled: *Objects and Method of Diet Adjustment in Diabetes*. Although insulin had yet to be isolated, researchers knew that the pancreas was the site of pathology – injecting diabetic dogs with pancreatic extract could normalize blood sugar levels. Woodyatt realized that the problem in the diabetic lie solely in pancreatic dysfunction, resulting in an inability to utilize excessive carbohydrate. At the time, physician's often fasted diabetics until glucose disappeared from the urine, the idea being to "rest" the pancreas. A normal diet was then slowly reintroduced, usually with carbohydrates first. Unfortunately, the diabetics soon found themselves back where they started, with sugar building up to malevolent levels within the blood stream.

That fasting cleared the bloodstream of sugar made Woodyatt curious, inspiring him to ask a simple question: if fasting diabetic patients resort to burning their own fat, why not just provide fat through diet, keep the carbohydrates away, and keep the diabetic in the fasted state indefinitely? It was a simple proposal of exclusion. It was a question that perhaps should have been asked sooner, but at the time it was easy for researchers to get lost in the details. Big questions still lingered, the largest was the fate of dietary fat: it was not clear if fat could be converted directly into sugar. But Woodyatt refused to let the gaps in knowledge lead to a dead end – when a pathway was unknown, he let empirical, macro-evidence guide him.

In this case, he knew another group had already experimented with a high fat/low carb diet in diabetics with striking success – even if fat was able to be converted into glucose it really didn't matter, reasoned Woodyatt, something appeared to be blocking its conversion. He was formulating a hypothesis that had only lingered in and out of researcher's minds, but had never been concretely suggested. Once he wrote it down, it seemed obvious: *why not shift the ratio of the diet in favor of fat, this way the diabetic would be able to rest his pancreas, remove the excess sugar from his bloodstream, and utilize fat instead as an energy source.* The smoldering problems of insulin, carbohydrates, and blood sugar were removed from the equation.

He couldn't help chastising the medical community for their inflexible, dogmatic assumptions, isolating the problem as a tendency toward dietary groupthink: "the universal custom of thinking of the food supply simply as so much carbohydrate, so much protein, so much fat and so many calories without further analysis," wrote Woodyatt. The patient doesn't even have to be deprived, he reasoned, they could consume the same amount of total calories. In a single sentence Woodyatt toppled the monolithic view of diet. Now, because of him, diet was no longer viewed as a concrete pillar, now it was a column built from subcategories (carbohydrate, protein, and fat) that could be manipulated, shifted, and restacked in different combinations depending on the needs of the patient.

While Woodyatt was exposing fissures in dietary preconceptions, in the summer of 1921, three hundred and fifty miles north east of Chicago at the Mayo clinic in Rochester Minnesota, a doctor named Russell Wilder published three short paragraphs in *The Clinical Bulletin*. The letter described the same dietary epiphany as Woodyatt — maintaining the fasting state by replacing carbohydrates with fat – but Wilder imagined treating a different disease: epilepsy. "It has occurred to us that the benefit of Dr. Geyelin's procedure may be dependent on the ketonemia which must result from such fasts, and that possibly equally good results could be obtained if a ketonemia were produced by some other means," wrote Wilder. But Wilder had made an additional leap of logic.

Woodyatt had suggested the dietary protocol simply as a means to sidestep the impaired carbohydrate metabolism of diabetics. How fasting, or the dietary maintenance of fasting, worked to control seizures demanded another explanation. Wilder reasoned perhaps there was more to it – suggesting the ketones generated from the diet might be of unrecognized significance. After all, they were the single metabolic variable shared between the fasting state and a low/carb high/fat diet. Until now, researchers assumed ketones were nothing but unhealthy metabolic debris, but now, because of Wilder, that assumption was questioned. Perhaps it was ketones themselves that were pulling the metabolic levers inside the brain of fasting epileptics. Wilder was anxious to test his theory. "It is proposed, therefore, to try the effect of such *ketogenic diets* on a series of epileptics."

It's hard to quantify the influence that words have. Attaching a name to an idea converts it from an abstraction into something tangible and concrete. Wilder's naming of the "ketogenic diet" was to thrust it into the clinic, now it was real, now it was something that could be measured, tested, and prescribed.

Under the lamp of Woodyatt and Wilder's clarifying epiphanies, Dr. Mynie Peterman, a mayo clinic pediatrician, enthusiastically put Wilder's theoretical diet to a clinical test. First, he strictly defined the ketogenic diet to be tested, parceling it into one gram of protein per kilogram of the child's body weight, 10-15 grams of carbohydrates per day, and the remainder of the calories in fat. Next, he began recruiting epileptic patients and convincing them to try the strange protocol.

The scientific community was watching closely – they eagerly waited for the results. Once released, Peterman's report revealed the diet's effect was incredible. Most of the children, once racked with convulsions, experienced an immediate and powerful remission. They began to live normal lives. The price was minimal. Occasional a child became nauseated and vomited, and so Peterman found a little orange juice was an instant fix. But most transitioned to the new diet well and had few complaints.

The ketogenic diet, at first only a fragile theory, was working. While running his clinical trials Peterman noticed something else. Not only were the vast majority of kids either experiencing greatly diminished numbers of seizures, or free of them altogether, but there seemed to be a striking change in their character. Peterman noticed the children were "sleeping better, were less irritable, and displayed an increased interest and alertness." This was in sharp contrast to the pharmacological treatments that dulled and muted the children, as if a wet blanket was pulled over their brains.

The ketogenic diet, Peterman observed, lifted the fog. Peterman followed 37 children on the diet for 4 months up to two and a half years. All tallied, sixty percent of the children became seizure free, 34.5% were improved, and 5.5% were not improved. The ketogenic diet was a resounding success – undeniably better than phenobarbital and bromides.

While the newly débuted "ketogenic diet" was being studied at the Mayo clinic, doctors on the East coast were still deeply immersed in neurochemical transformation induced by fasting. Therapeutically, fasting had obvious limitations. The biggest problem, doctors realized, is that fasting was clearly only a temporary solution. The seizures were greatly diminished, if not stopped altogether while the child was not eating, but of course, it could not be maintained. In some of the more mild cases, after the fast, the seizures never returned. But in many cases, once the child resumed eating, the seizures gradually resumed. Wilder's ketogenic diet offered an immediate solution to this problem. The therapeutic effect of fasting could now be extended on a patient by patient basis.

News from the Mayo clinic trial quickly spread. Massachusetts General Hospital, in 1924, pivoted away from fasting and adopted the ketogenic diet as a treatment for epilepsy. Others were soon to follow. New studies tallied similar results as the original done by Peterman, and others also noticed the positive effects the diet seemed to have on the children, one researcher commented, "the diet is well tolerated without causing any untoward symptoms in the patients. On the contrary, they seem to be more alert and less nervous." After tinkering with the ratios, clinicians determined that a formula of 4 parts fat to 1 part protein/carbohydrate seemed to work best (a ratio that has stood the test of time and today is known as the *classic ketogenic diet.*)

Instructions for the ketogenic diet, meal plans, and extensive tables listing the nutritional composition of foods were added to textbooks. In response to rising demand, the Mayo Clinic published a pamphlet describing detailed meal plans and recipes for the ketogenic diet. Soon clinicians and dietitians at hospitals across the county were prescribing the new dietary treatment for epilepsy. Untold numbers of families with epileptic children were restocking their pantries and adjusting their family dinners. For doctors, and the families of the afflicted, it was probably an easy choice, the only two drugs on the market were highly sedative, and the diet was the opposite; it required some work, it wasn't an easy fix, but the benefit was striking, immediate, and enduring for most. Word swiftly spread and the ketogenic diet became the preferred therapy for epilepsy across the country. "The results of fasting and the ketogenic diet are apparently the best that are obtained by any therapeutic procedure that we have to offer the epileptics in childhood today," Geyelin told the American College of Physicians at a gathering in New Orleans in 1928.

"Like Stones for a Mosaic"

Charles Howland refused to give up. In 1922, undeterred by his brother and Gamble's failure to find a definitive answer, he set out to expand the list of experts to help answer his question. He singled out Dr. Stanley Cobb, the associate professor of neuropathology at Harvard Medical School. Cobb was a cautious and careful scientist from a prominent Boston family that was speculated to have entered the neurosciences as a result of a childhood stammer. Cobb was already familiar with Howland's story – he was in the audience a year earlier when Geyelin presented the case of his young cousin's trek to Battle Creek and the successful treatment by Conklin.

To Cobb, the story was not entirely surprising. Rumors of Conklin's early results had intrigued him, and he had begun to investigate fasting's effect within his own lab. When Geyelin had finished his presentation, Cobb excitedly shared his own work with the attendees, commenting that he had witnessed the therapeutic effect first-hand – preventing convulsions in animals by fasting them. What *did* surprise Cobb, however, was that now, one year later, the father of the child Geyelin spoke of was standing in his office, and asking for his help. Cobb had revealed how he felt about Conklin's work in an earlier conversation with a colleague when he stated that fasting treatment was significant because it "revealed the relationship between epilepsy and metabolism." In Cobb's mind, this relationship demanded to be explored. Cobb agreed to help. Howland scribbled out a check for enough to fund Cobb's efforts for two years.

Cobb knew the difficulty of what he had just signed up for. He would have to tap the same dogged grit that allowed him to overcome his childhood stammer. To get to the bottom of Howland's question was to step into the unknown – despite Gamble's intense effort, few solid leads had been found – all that was known for sure was fasting worked. Instinctually, he knew he would need help.

First on Cobb's list to conscript into the effort was a Harvard educated doctor named William Lennox. Enthusiastic, innovative, and bold, Lennox became interested in epilepsy after witnessing the unrelenting and mysterious convulsions of a friend's daughter while studying the health of missionary families in China in 1917. The strange nature of the disease stirred something in Lennox. In a stroke of serendipity, Lennox happened to be visiting Boston in the spring of 1921 and attended the AMA meeting where Geyelin presented. Suddenly, Lennox found himself at a turning point. He commented that he was "thrilled by Geyelin's demonstration and having a compelling interest in epilepsy and its treatment, my missionary zeal was abruptly transferred from Chinese to epilepsy," The timing was perfect – infused with Howland's cash, Cobb offered Lennox a position. It didn't take much convincing from Cobb to recruit Lennox. The intense curiosity simmering inside him made the decision easy.

Together they launched into the problem. Howland's question was now expanded to include the ketogenic diet that had been defined a year earlier by Wilder. The diet was the preservation of the fasting state, and so by extension, the same rules probably applied. Whatever mechanism fasting worked through to mitigate seizures was most likely the same for the ketogenic diet. Wilder had added another suspect to the lineup: ketone bodies. Like Gamble, Cobb and Lennox dove into the metabolic transformation that occurred within fasting epileptic patients with painstaking detail. And like Gamble, after some time had passed, they realized the answer was not going to present itself easily. Strangely, it seemed every path they followed ended with a contradiction – as if they were purposefully being toyed with.

For example, Geyelin had noticed his fasting patients excreted acid – the more acid excreted, the fewer seizures. Ketones are acidic, so maybe, they reasoned, it was the increase in acidosis within the patient's blood plasma from ketosis that was somehow acting to slow seizures. Other clues led them in this direction. Acidifying the patient's plasma by injecting acid directly into their veins seemed to have an anti-seizure effect. But the problem was in the timing.

The anti-seizure effect didn't exactly track the acidification – once the pH level was made acidic, it took a while for the seizures to slow. Similarly, when the blood pH level was returned to normal, it took some time for the seizures to return. This didn't match with the fact the induction of ketosis, either by fasting or the ketogenic diet, typically resulted in an immediate reduction in seizures – so clearly it wasn't the acidity alone that mattered. Also, when they acidified the patients' blood, their seizures eventually slowed, but then after a period of time, even while the blood was kept acidic, the seizures would roar back with vicious ferocity, as if a damn had been burst.

Maybe, as Wilder suggested, it was the ketone bodies themselves? To test this idea Lennox and Cobb put a patient on the ketogenic diet. Once her seizures stopped, she was injected with bi-carbonate (a compound that counteracts acid). When they tested her blood after the injection of bi-carbonate, surprisingly, there was an increase in ketone bodies, but, even with the increased ketones, her seizures returned with a vengeance – so clearly it wasn't the ketone bodies by themselves. Every time they tried to isolate the relevant variable it would slip just out of reach.

The nature of the problem was not lost on Cobb and Lennox. They recognized what it was: an incredibly complex and interrelated series of neurochemical alterations. The search, they realized, was probably just getting started: "The painstaking accumulation of apparently unrelated facts must go on," wrote Lennox, "until, like stones for a mosaic, they are sufficient in number to permit their assembly into a complete and intelligible design." The answer remained a map of the world before Columbus. The yet-to-be-explored forbade a complete image. And the existing technology was too rudimentary for the time being to fill in the gaps. Howland's question, it appeared, like the mapping of the earth, might be a multigenerational effort.

"Them Thar Hills"

Even if Cobb and Lennox failed to find a clear, succinct answer to Howland's question, something special was happening in Boston. In 1930, Cobb, now 44 years old, was appointed Director of the newly formed neurological unit at Boston City Hospital. Under his Directorship, a powerhouse team of researchers, all united by an intense interest in epilepsy, fortuitously fell into place. Lennox followed Cobb to Boston City Hospital and they were soon joined by a Harvard trained neurosurgeon named Tracy Putnam and a John's Hopkins trained neurologist, Houston Merritt. Putnam and Merritt met while in the throes of a neurological internship at the hospital and they experienced a powerful connection, forming a deep and enduring friendship. Both were described as "brilliant" and capable of having "unusual insights."

Putman had more than a professional interest in epilepsy because two of his relatives – one a cousin whom he regarded as a sister – suffered from the affliction. Their talent, passion and intellect did not go unnoticed by Cobb, he actively recruited them into the research effort. Together the group formed a tempest of creativity. What happened at Boston City Hospital was a rare alignment of the stars, a group of personalities that collectively elevated their work far beyond any single individual's ability. An uninhibited atmosphere of infectious enthusiasm encouraged bold ideas. A writer described the unit: "its roster establishes the unit among the greatest institutions ever of its kind."

But the timing couldn't have been worse. The fragile realization of the extraordinary research team was almost shattered in its infancy. When the great depression struck in 1930, it crushed research programs across the country. For Cobb and Lennox, when Howland's cash ran out, Harvard rushed to form an "Epilepsy Commission" so their work wouldn't die on the vine. The program was funded by voluntary donations – which shut off like a spigot in the aftermath of Black Tuesday. At the last second, the Rockefeller institute stepped in – if they hadn't, the history of epilepsy treatment may have had its course altered in incalculable ways.

The group knew the largest obstacle to understanding and improving treatments was a lack of good animal models to study. The current models used chemicals to induce seizures – a clumsy and inconsistent method that gave sometimes wildly different results. The newly developed electroencephalographic (EEG) instrument was able to record electrical discharge from patient's brains. When strapped to an epileptic patient's head, through a frantic amplification of squiggles on paper, the machine revealed a tornado of excessive electrical discharge.

No one knew why the storm occurred, where it came from, or what caused it to disappear, but the new machine identified what a seizure was: electrical impulses firing without purpose – an overload of signal pulsating through the brain. Putnam reasoned that if a seizure was an electrical discharge then maybe he could trigger a seizure in animals by the same route: by administering an electric shock. The group seized Putnam's insight. Using parts from an electric motor taken from a salvaged WWI German airplane, they assembled a makeshift machine that would meter out a trigger – a measured electric shock.

After some deliberation, Putman and Merritt decided to test their new machine on cats. The idea was simple: test the cats to see how much of a pulse caused them to have a seizure, then, give the same cats the drug to be tested, wait two hours, and repeat the test. If the cats required more of a shock to trigger a seizure while on the drug, then it was logical to assume the drug was anti-convulsive. Testing known drugs confirmed their logic. When the cats were given bromide it took 50% more current to generate a seizure than before; when given phenobarbital, it took three to four times more current than before. Their model was consistent and reproducible.

The group then made a vital observation. Ever since the discovery of bromides it had always been assumed it was the hypnotic or sedative effect of drugs that muted convulsions – the two properties were inseparable. The new experimental system allowed them to test that assumption. When Putman and Merritt drugged the cats with bromide and phenobarbital to the exact same sedative-state – to the point that prevented the cats from walking – and then used their apparatus to test the seizure threshold – phenobarbital was still much better. This teased out a critical detail. It implied that the sedative property and the anti-convulsive property were not chained together, they could be separated.

They now realized it wasn't necessarily the sedative property of the drugs that made them work. This discovery unshackled the search for new anti-seizure drugs; effectively it removed a massive barrier that had inhibited anti-seizure drug development for about seventy years. The narrow canyon researchers were searching in was suddenly expanded into an open field.

Putnam and Merritt realized the opportunity and began to use their animal model to test new drugs. As modest as it seems on the surface, the experimental system was revolutionary. This was one of the first scaled-up uses of animals to test drugs that might prove useful in humans, a process now called *translational medicine*. Given that phenobarbital was the best drug available, Putnam made a short leap of logic; he would test derivatives of phenobarbital –compounds that were chemically similar. Their animal model, and method of screening compounds, was Henry Ford's newly developed assembly-line recapitulated into the industry of drug discovery – a quantum leap in productivity. Before the process of drug discovery was mostly accidental, now it was *purposeful*. The system vastly streamlined the probability for successfully finding new drugs because it allowed for screening *en masse* – they would be able to churn through chemicals with untold speed and precision.

Putnam began to search. He combed through the Eastman Chemical company catalog looking for compounds that were structurally just a shade away from phenobarbital. At the same time, he was calling pharmaceutical companies, asking if they had anything that resembled phenobarbital. Specifically, because they had shown the hypnotic quality of anti-seizure drugs was not essential, he requested "compounds that were thought to be hypnotic but had not proven to be." Only one returned Putnam's call, Author Dox, a chemist at Parke-Davis.

At the end of April a package arrived at Boston City Hospital from Dox with Putnam's name on it. Inside, were 7 analogs of phenobarbital and a dozen other compounds that fit Putnam's description. Dox warned Putnam of the futility of what he was trying to accomplish. He told him his search was "a waste of time, because the compounds had already been thoroughly tested and were inactive." But Dox had only tested the compounds for the sedative effect, assuming, like everyone, that was enough to rule them out as anticonvulsive drugs. He was unaware that the Boston group had reason to believe otherwise.

One of the phenobarbital derivatives, called phenytoin, had been sitting on the shelf at Parke-Davis for decades. The company had purchased the compound from a German organic chemist in 1908 hoping it had sedative properties. But when the compound was found to be only mildly sedative it was placed on the shelf in a store room and forgotten. The overlooked compound was first on the list for Putnam and Merritt to test. They knew it had failed as a sleeping pill, and so had less of a sedative effect than current drugs. When they gave the drug to the cats it was clear they weren't overly impaired; Dox was right, it was only mildly sedative. But when they tested the cat's seizure threshold it left them in astonishment. The drug raised the threshold far beyond the other known drugs, *without heavily sedating them*. This was exactly what they were looking for, the holy grail of epilepsy treatment, a drug that was less sedative yet powerfully anticonvulsive.

The early 1930's were a much different time. Regulators didn't require preclinical safety testing for new drugs (the Food, Drug, and Cosmetic Act was signed in 1938). Nevertheless, just to be sure, Putnam and Merritt handed the drug over to a toxicologist at Harvard, and one at Parke-Davis. Both found phenytoin could be given to cats, dogs, and rats at very high single and repeated doses without immediate toxic effects. This was enough to clear the path and they started treating patients in May.

By the summer of 1938 they had treated 200 adult and pediatric patients with phenytoin, now branded Dilantin, and presented their results at an AMA meeting in San Francisco. The results were remarkable. According to Putnam and Merritt, Dilantin was able to eliminate, or greatly reduce the seizures in 85% of the patients tested. Minor toxic symptoms were reported in 15% of the patients and "more serious toxic reactions" were reported in 5%. Six days later, Parke-Davis added Dilantin to its list of marketed products.

The rest is history. The popularity of the drug grew quickly. By 1940 it was hailed as ushering in a new epoch in the treatment of epilepsy. One doctor called it, "the most remarkable and important chemotherapeutic agent in the convulsive disorders since 1912..." Truly a new era had taken hold for epileptic patients. Across the country, doctors began prescribing Dilantin as a first line treatment for their patients.

The discovery of Dilantin did something else: it aroused and unbridled the capitalistic instinct of pharmaceutical companies. They paid close attention to the discovery of Dilantin. Perhaps even more important than the discovery of Dilantin itself, was the permanent enshrinement of the methodology established by Putnam and Merritt. The significance of Putnam and Merritt's animal model was not lost on big-pharma. The companies quickly established their own in-house large scale drug screening programs. Putnam and Merritt themselves screened over 700 compounds for anti-convulsive activity between 1937 and 1945. The massively scaled-up efforts produced results. Over the next two decades, a dozen new anticonvulsants hit the shelves at the pharmacy.

As quickly as the new era of anticonvulsive drugs was ushered in, the ketogenic diet was ushered out. Dilantin was viewed as modern medicine at its best. It was a symbol of progress, mankind's continuous vector of medical advancement. With the advent of seizure control for many patients in the form of a pill, the onerous diet was soon regarded as "rigid and expensive", and began a sharp decent from favor. A pill was so much easier. A pill took a doctor seconds to scribble its prescription. The diet took the time and effort of many individuals; the doctor, a dietitian, nurses, and the families. With a pill, everyone was *released*. They no longer had to plan every shopping list and meal. The kids and families could live normal lives. They no longer were cast as outsiders. They could enjoy the same food everybody else was having. They could now have birthday cake, pancakes with syrup, and dessert alongside their friends and family – they didn't have to watch from the sidelines.

History is full of research that drifts off like an unfinished conversation. Alongside the ketogenic diet, Howland's original question faded from relevance. It was a strange query from a by-gone era. How fasting, or the ketogenic diet worked to stop seizures no longer mattered to the vast majority of researchers. But not everyone felt that way. It faded from view with a smattering of unheard protest. At the Mayo clinic, Peterman, found Dilantin "disappointing" compared to the ketogenic diet. Ironically, years later, speaking to a group of resident physicians at the NIH (National Institute of Health, Washington D.C.), Dr. Merritt was rumored to tell the young doctors that his discovery of phenytoin was a major setback to the understanding of epilepsy.

He felt the line of research started by Howland's original question of why fasting worked, and then morphing to the ketogenic diet, was a thread that could have ultimately led to a deeper understanding into the mechanisms of epilepsy. In 1960, almost 40 years after he was recruited to work on Howland's question, Lennox looked back nostalgically, "Though interest in fasting (or the ketogenic diet) as a treatment has almost vanished, doubtless much scientific gold remains in them thar hills".

By 1990, the ketogenic diet was all but completely forgotten. It was a strange, antiquated side-note that most physicians felt belonged in a history book, not a modern textbook. The diet was labeled "rigid, unpalatable, and constraining on daily life." Johns Hopkins, one of the original hospitals to help develop and utilize the diet in the 20's and 30's, barely managed to preserve a single prescribing physician – Dr. John Freeman, and his dietitian, Millicent Kelly, a seventy-two year old that had been administering the diet for forty years. There was vanishingly little demand for their services. Kelly taught the ketogenic diet to the families of less than 10 children a year. To the doctors around the country, Freeman and Kelly might as well have been a museum exhibit.

Kelly scribbled in an old notepad, calculating ratios and jotting down recipes for the families. "Together, we were the keepers of the flame," Freeman later wrote. Besides Kelly, so few dietitians were trained in the nuances of the diet that when it was used, it was administered sloppily, and the children often had bad outcomes. The lessons of the past, that it took precise calculations to achieve the best seizure control, were all but lost. The bad results were folded into the perception that the diet was old, outdated, and not as effective as the current drugs. The widespread opinion was that the diet "did not work and was difficult to tolerate" and its use was "no longer justified." Across the country, its use became almost nonexistent.

"Wait a Minute, This Didn't Have to Happen"

As the Abrahamses flew to Baltimore for the last remaining chance to treat Charlie's unremitting seizures, their thoughts cartwheeled between sadness, desperation, and the last sliver of hope. Most likely they were experiencing the same emotions as the Howlands as they rode the train toward Battle Creek eighty years earlier. As he traversed the American landscape, Abrahams was entirely unaware of the rich history surrounding the ketogenic diet as a treatment for epilepsy. That it was once the standard-of-care for epilepsy would have shocked and bewildered him even more so. For Abrahams, and most doctors and patients across the country, the ketogenic diet was *dead* – reduced to the equivalent of an herbalist working out of a strip mall.

When they arrived at Johns Hopkins they met with Dr. Freeman and his dietitian, Millicent Kelly. The pair seemed perfectly matched. Dr. Freeman was the maverick. "He was larger than life; fearless; he knew he was considered an outlier by a lot of his colleagues, but in a way I think that intrigued him." Millicent was the soft side – comforting, Grandmother-like mannerisms that were amplified to almost cartoonish levels. With a charming and soothing voice that seemed to round the edges of every word, she explained the diet to Abrahams. With no time to spare, they began the diet with a jump start, they fasted Charlie the rest of the day and into the next.

By the next day, when Abrahams held his son he could already tell a difference; he just felt "less intense", like something had been turned down. By the next day, forty-eight hours later, something remarkable happened: his son stopped having seizures. *Completely.* The Abrahamses returned home brimming with optimism and hope. Days passed, and then weeks, and the seizures remained at bay. The diet had an incredibly powerful impact. It had done what of drugs and surgery were unable to do; it had brought his son back from the abyss. Charlie began to thrive. His mental capacity and energy returned. The house, once filled with tears, was now filled with joy.

The story of the Abrahamses would have ended there – they would have been just one of the ten or so that Dr. Freeman and Millicent quietly helped every year. But like Howland before him, the experience aroused something deep. Medicine had failed them. Things begin to stir in

Abrahams when he returned to his normal life. Something just didn't sit well. "All of a sudden my eyes opened up in the middle of the night, and I said 'wait a minute, this didn't have to happen.' Ninety percent of these seizures didn't have to occur. Waking up around the clock, and pouring drugs down his throat, didn't have to occur." Abrahams' epiphany morphed into puzzlement and anger. What motivated him the most is that he was in a position to prevent this from happening to others.

Where Howland had the money of a wealthy corporate lawyer, Abrahams had something even better – perhaps the best resource in the world for taking up a cause: Hollywood. Abrahams had produced blockbuster hits like Airplane, Naked Gun, and Hot Shots. If it was simply a lack of information, he could change that. So he and his wife Nancy started the now famous Charlie Foundation dedicated to disseminating information about the ketogenic diet so Charlie's story would not be repeated. On October 26th, 1994, the NBC news program Dateline brought Charlie's story into millions of living rooms across the country.

At the end of the show viewers were given a number to call. Families that called were sent a video from the Charlie Foundation titled *An Introduction to the Ketogenic Diet*. The foundation also mailed the same tape to neurologists throughout the country. Shortly after, neurologists were mailed another video titled *The Ketogenic Diet: Doctors Version*. It was a well-orchestrated plan and its impact was enormous. Abrahams also had the Charlie foundation ready to fund a seven-center trial designed to measure the impact of the ketogenic diet once and for all. A trial would serve to demonstrate the efficacy of the forgotten diet for both patients and doctors.

It was timed perfectly. Shortly before the Dateline special the Charlie Foundation quietly had doctors, dietitians, nurses, and families with an epileptic child come to Johns Hopkins and receive intensive training on the use of the proven Johns Hopkins ketogenic diet protocol. The doctors and their staffs were then ready and waiting for the anticipated surge of new patients coming from media blitz that began with the prime-time Dateline special. As expected, the kids came from all corners of the country, desperate to try the new diet. Four years later Freeman published the results from 150 kids that entered the trial. The patient group enrolled in the trial was a tough lot.

As a group, they averaged 410 seizures per month and had already failed to improve after trying an average of 6.2 medications. Nevertheless, the outcome was dramatic. Of the 55% still on the diet after a year, 27% were close to seizure free, 23% were significantly improved, and the remaining 5% had a less than 50% reduction of seizures. Three to six years later, 27% of these same children had few to no seizures and most were off of the diet and on fewer to no medication. To further raise public awareness, a year before the data from the trial was published, Abrahams released an ABC television movie titled *First Do No Harm* starring his good friend Meryl Streep. It was the dramatic portrayal of a Midwestern family's struggle to find the ketogenic diet for their child with severe and unresponsive epilepsy. Eight million viewers watched the movie the night it was aired.

In truth, the Charlie Foundation's clinical trial just confirmed the results of the thirteen other studies that had been performed since Wilder first purposed the diet as a treatment in 1921. The only difference this time, because of Jim Abrahams' elegantly choreographed media campaign, people were paying attention. The study was presented at the annual American Epilepsy Society in 1996. Before the study was presented, the ketogenic diet was almost never mentioned at the annual gathering. But this time, combined with the media firestorm, it precipitated an avalanche of research the following year, and only grew in the years after that. The ketogenic diet had been resurrected – as quickly as it had fallen, because of the discovery of Dilantin, it had been revived by a passionate family and their sick child.

––––––––

Seven minutes and fifty-five seconds into the Dateline special featuring Charlie's story, Charlie's doctor, Donald Shields, said something important. The reporter asked Dr. Shields: "You had some knowledge this diet was probably working back at Johns Hopkins (Dr. Shields and Dr. Freeman were actually good friends), yet you dissuaded the Abrahams from attempting it, how come?" Dr. Shields paused, looked at the ceiling, and said, "Well, because I don't think we had exhausted all of the medical approaches yet. There were actually other medications we hadn't tried yet." Drawing a distinction between so called "medical approaches" and the ketogenic diet reveals volumes of the way many doctors view the dietary protocol – something existing outside of the realm of real medicine – something strange, nonconventional, and alternative. Why else would the diet have faded into complete obscurity in the first place?

Even today the diet is rarely used as a first line treatment. It is still something held in reserve. Epilepsy is almost always treated first with drugs. Medication will make half of the patient's seizure free for an extended period of time. But if a patient doesn't respond to the first drug the odds rapidly diminish. In these cases a second drug will only make an additional 14% seizure free. If that drug fails then the likelihood of seizure control using drugs falls to about 1 to 2 percent. Remarkably, even with the most recent anti-seizure drugs, these ratios have remained essentially the same throughout the century– as if some fundamental barrier cannot be breached by drugs alone. So that leaves more than 30% of epileptic patients without seizure control even with the latest, and best medications.

Before Abrahams pulled the diet from obscurity, these patients had nowhere to turn. Today, this is where the ketogenic diet is typically used – as an option of last resort. For the over 30% of patients with uncontrolled seizures after failing drug therapy the ketogenic diet is a godsend. If maintained properly, it renders half of this desperate group either completely or extremely close to seizure free. These incredible results have been shown consistently in study after study throughout the 20th century. In addition, most kids who use the diet can transition back to a normal western diet after two years, never need drugs again, and remain seizure free.

After combing through the statistics an inevitable question arises: why is the diet only held as an option of last resort? One can't help but wonder: which is better as a first-line treatment, drugs, or the ketogenic diet? To be sure, the comparisons, from trials alone, are not apples to apples. A direct head to head comparison has never been done. The answer to this question remains unknown.

However, there is a very important difference between the studies of anti-seizure drugs and the ketogenic diet: all of the modern studies of the ketogenic diet use a patient population that has failed drug treatment. The dietary trials have a built-in bias from the starting line. The tests done on the ketogenic diet are enrolled with the hardest cases – patients with gritty, embedded seizures that refuse to be blunted by the best medications available. "You've already peeled off the easiest cases. It's like running a one-hundred yard dash with a weight chained to your leg," said Dr. James Wheless, a pediatric neurologist, and a recognized expert on the use of the ketogenic diet. Even in the face of such difficult odds, the ketogenic diet shows incredible results.

Of course, any comparison of diet verses drugs must also include side effects. Even modern drugs aren't completely benign. When Charlie was saturated in anti-seizure drugs Abrahams described him as a "zombie who lived in his car seat." Although technology has continued to separate the sedative effect and the anti-seizure effect, it is not perfect. Drugs often leave patients lethargic, dizzy, and with double vision. Rashes appear, weight gain, abnormal liver function, kidney stones, and constipation.

The biggest difference between anti-seizure medication and the ketogenic diet occurs in the brain. Indeed, the brain is ground zero in the debate of diet versus drugs. The side effects that occur from medication are not there in the diet, in fact, the opposite occurs. Doctors today notice the same mental effects as the original pioneers of the diet back at the beginning of the 20th century: increased alertness, improved behavior, reduced anxiety and depression. How the patient experiences life is markedly different between drugs and the diet – a variable that defies quantification.

The strict form of the diet is not without some issues. Side effects do occur, but they are very minor, including changes in lipid profiles, kidney stones, constipation, and a subtle slowing of growth. However, improvements in the diet formulation, macronutrient sources, supplements, and interventions have greatly diminished lipid abnormalities, constipation and kidney stones.

A 2010 study at Johns Hopkins followed the outcomes of children treated with the ketogenic diet from 1993 to 2008 and found almost no long-term adverse effects. The only obvious effect was growth. Height was found to be reduced by 5 cm from the *expected* average. All other laboratory values were normal. Most importantly, the study found the subjects had continued to either maintain, or improve on seizure control, even into adulthood. Most of the families had few regrets and would recommend the diet to others. All added up – results combined with side-effects – many experts in the field give a nod to the ketogenic diet when directly compared to drugs. They feel the diet is often simply the best medical option. "No anticonvulsive drugs have that rate of beneficial effect," wrote Dr. Freeman.

Despite the heroic efforts of Abrahams, his wife Nancy, and the Charlie Foundation, the ketogenic diet is still today underutilized. When an epileptic child enters a neurologist's practice the typical scenario goes like this: the patient is prescribed a first-line drug. As stated above, this works about half of the time. For the half that fail to respond, the neurologist will prescribe another drug. This time the drug works in about one in seven kids (it doesn't matter which drug is chosen, the statistics remain the same). For the kids that don't respond to the second drug the neurologist will now almost always try a third. The chance the third drug will work now falls to one percent. This leaves over one in three kids that come back to the neurologist office in a desperate situation, after having failed three drugs. The neurologist now has a decision to make. According to a 2008 special report issued by a consortium of 26 world-recognized experts using the ketogenic diet from nine countries, this is precisely where the diet should be prescribed, after the failure of two to three drugs.

At this point the data begs to be heard: the ketogenic diet will make over half of this desperate group of kids either entirely, or very close to seizure free – the other half simply can't or won't maintain the diet for a variety of reasons – either they find the diet isn't working, or it's too hard to maintain. Prescribing a fourth drug has a vanishingly small chance of working. Yet, strangely, in many cases, the neurologist will keep going; writing script after script for more and more drugs – many never suggesting the diet – the same dreadful place Charlie and his family found themselves.

When I asked Jim if Charlie's "story" still happens today, he responded in a sober tone: "Sadly, Yes. And in many ways its worse; the reason is because there are more drugs. The physicians frequently say, 'well there is another drug, let's try that instead.' From what we see, from those who contact us, I don't know the exact statics, but rarely is the diet prescribed after the failure of two or three medications." Why the diet continues to be marginalized is a poignant question. "It's a culture shift," said Dr. Wheless. "The mindset today is to take a pill and be done. If the diet was in pill form it would be the best treatment available."

It raises an important question. Are we as a culture, both patients and physicians, willing to marginalize an incredibly effective therapy at the expense of some convenience? The question is especially relevant considering the price paid is so incredibly high. "One of the things that pisses me off the most is that the whole degree of difficulty thing; it's not a medical question," said Abrahams. "When you're holding your kid while he has hundreds of seizures a day, and then you find out doctors aren't giving you all the information...because they think, 'it's too difficult' – where in medical school did they teach a course on what's considered too difficult for the parents of a critically ill child."

To get this right is not trivial. Epilepsy affects 65 million people across the globe – almost one percent of the world's population. The most updated statistic released by the CDC claim 1 in 26 people will develop epilepsy at some point in their life. Despite extensive testing, over half of all cases are idiopathic, meaning no reason for the illness can be found. It mostly affects children, but can also affect adults – the chances increasing with age. It is a terrifying disease because there are so many unknowns.

Still today, after centuries of investigation, researchers cannot tell you exactly what a seizure is, where it comes from, or why it stops. Words crop up like "multifactorial", and "network effect"; which, although true, are really a way of saying "we don't know exactly" – a bucket to throw very difficult problems in. Epilepsy erodes at the edges of life, interrupting, stealing, and isolating its victims. It is not passive. Over time, if severe enough, epilepsy won't allow the brain to develop correctly. It is a tremendous burden for societies across the globe. And to let an extraordinary therapy remain under prescribed because of an undefined apathy is tragic and deserves an explanation.

Near the end of the Dateline special featuring Charlies story, the reporter asked Dr. Shields a final question: "Dr. Freeman tells us that fifty to seventy percent of the patients that come through his doors and get put on the ketogenic diet have success. Can you think of any drugs, in these hard cases, that have fifty to seventy percent success rates?" Dr. Shield's again looked to the ceiling before answering, "Probably not anything that comes up to that level." After some reflection, Dr. Shields backpedaled, and came up with a possible explanation for this astonishing situation – a reason why the diet is so often ignored. "There is no big drug company behind the ketogenic diet.

And there will never be unless somebody starts marketing sausage and eggs with cream sauce on it as a drug." Abrahams agrees with Dr. Shield's assessment about why the diet remains in the shadows, "It's not in the form of a pill, it can't be administered with a scalpel, and the only people who profit from the ketogenic diet are the patients," said Abrahams.

At the front-line of the Charlie Foundation's efforts is their head nutritionist Beth Zupec-Kania. Over her 24 years with the Charlie Foundation Beth has trained dietitians in 10 countries and treated thousands of epileptic patients around the world. Perhaps more than anyone, she has witnessed the power of the ketogenic diet to treat epilepsy first hand. Typically, when she sees a patient they are on at least two anti-seizure drugs, have failed many more, are sick, frustrated, and exhausted. The patients that finally turn to the diet do so for more than one reason, said Zupec-Kania, "Their seizures continue unabated, or they are experiencing such severe side-effects that they are essentially nonfunctional, or both. Sadly, it's *usually both*." Most are left simmering in a state of pronounced lethargy because of the drugs.

Some drugs are worse than others. "The worst drug is Topamax", said Zupec-Kania. "The nickname that the doctors call it behind the backs of patients is 'Dope-a-max' because it makes you feel so dopey. The patients can't think of words that they used to know." With the diet, she says that parents often notice a marked mental improvement once the child achieves ketosis. And this improvement occurs *while the patients are on the same amount of drugs*. Neurologists typically won't start reducing the drugs until the patient has maintained the diet for at least a month; after it's clear they are tolerating it well. The difference is striking. "All of a sudden the kid is paying attention, or stringing words together, kind of coming out of a fog," said Zupec-Kania. "Jim has a video of this mom describing her six year old son: 'he got up, he went to the bathroom, he cleaned up, and he came back to bed, and he hadn't done that in the past year.' The moment he went into ketosis he got his life back."

Zupec-Kania said the short term side effects from the diet are preventable and researchers have yet to find any long term side effects. In fact, she has a different take. "I think these patients are healthier because of what they are not eating. Having worked with thousands of people, many of them will continue leaving processed foods and sugar out of their diets and are healthier in the long run," she says. Through her quarter century of experience she has also made another striking observation.

The ridged boundaries of the diet, the 4 to 1 ratio that has been the 'gold standard' for patients, may not be as vital to achieving seizure control as once thought. "Lots of patients probably don't need the full blown ketogenic diet to get better; we could probably use something far more liberal and have the same effect. And I'm not even talking about the Modified Atkins Diet (which is used mainly for adolescents and adults with epilepsy), I'm talking about a paleo-type diet. I spoke to a mom last night who said her son just started having seizures out of the blue and after her nutritionist eliminated wheat and sugar from his diet his seizures stopped immediately. I would love to spare some people of the difficulty of the rigid form of the diet if it's not needed. And now we're finding just a low glycemic index diet can work in some cases. There is a whole spectrum of people and a whole spectrum of diets to meet their needs.

Dr. Jung Rho, of the University of Calgary is on the forefront of the current effort to answer Howland's original question. For Rho, the question remains as haunting today as it did in 1921. Rho is nearing the end of a $2 million dollar, five year grant from the NIH to find the mechanism behind the ketogenic diet's action on epilepsy. And as with those that came before him – Cobb, Lennox, Gamble, and Dr. Howland –the answer, wrote Rho, "remains elusive". Rho's estimation of the diet's effect is essentially the same as Lennox's *"stones forming a mosaic"* description almost a century ago: "At present, there are many hypotheses regarding KD (ketogenic diet) action, and while each is uniquely compelling, it is becoming more apparent that the KD likely works through multiple mechanisms," wrote Rho.

It's not surprising Rho and others have yet to pin down the diet's exact mechanism-of-action, given the nature of the human brain; an organ with 125 trillion neural synapses just in the cerebral cortex alone, a number roughly equal to the number of stars in 1,500 Milky Way galaxies. That level of staggering complexity, combined with the fact the pathophysiological mechanism behind seizures is still largely unknown, appears to have rendered Howland's question *still* out of our technological reach. Perhaps the most important realization from Rho's research is a deeper understanding of the nature of epilepsy: "The scientific literature involving the KD strongly supports the notion that epilepsy may indeed in part represent a "metabolic disease", and that this concept could serve as a novel framework for the development of more effective anti-seizure drugs," wrote Rho in July of 2015.

"The Genie is Out of the Bottle"

Even though, within the largely incentive driven arena of medicine, the ketogenic diet is still clearly under-prescribed today as a therapy for epilepsy, Jim Abrahams single-handedly managed to thrust the forgotten therapy back into the public and scientific consciousness. Before his Hollywood fueled campaign, the diet lie dormant – an artifact – after, researchers were once again stirred by the curious power of the ketogenic diet. Jim unknowingly resurrected a query from a by-gone era. To any curious biochemist, it is *still* astonishing in its own right that a simple shift in macromolecular consumption could have such a profound effect on brain chemistry.

By the late 1990's, researchers turned their attention and laboratory space over to the ketogenic diet with revolutionary zeal. The number of researcher papers containing the phrase "ketogenic diet" exploded – from only two-hundred and twenty-five before the year 2000, to one-thousand four-hundred in the fifteen years after the year 2000. The earlier articles published were almost exclusively about the role of the diet in epilepsy, but around the turn of the century researchers had begun to nudge at the margins of the diet, exploring its possible role beyond epilepsy. Researchers, for the first time, began asking other questions of the diet: could it be used to treat or prevent other diseases?

First it was cancer in 1995. It was a tiny study – only two little girls with brain cancer – but the results hinted at a potent impact and precipitated an avalanche of research into ketosis and cancer. As biochemists uncovered the unique mechanistic-details of ketosis it opened new possibilities. One paper, in 2003, by NIH scientist Richard Veech and George Cahill, was a siren call.

Specifically, it suggested the ketogenic diet, or ketone bodies by themselves, had the potential to affect a wide swath of pathologic conditions precipitated by insulin resistance and dysfunctional mitochondrial metabolism – fundamental processes that can lead to a constellation of problems. "What are the potential uses of beta-hydroxybutyrate in addition to pediatric epilepsy?" asked Veech, "Theoretically, any condition wherein oxygen supply to cells may be limited is an avenue for investigation. The list would encompass almost every disease state." The paper was a foot in the door, behind which was an open-ended spectrum of possibility.

Other researchers took notice. Studies on physical performance, Alzheimer's, and depression began in 2004. Parkinson's disease, traumatic brain injury, type 2 diabetes, Lafora body disease, polycystic ovary syndrome (PCOS), and metabolic syndrome in 2005, amyotrophic lateral sclerosis (ALS or Lou Gehrig's disease) in 2006, nonalcoholic fatty liver disease in 2007.

Incredibly, perhaps counterintuitively, the ketogenic diet showed promise to "modify" the course of one disease after the next. The strangely vast spectrum of diseases the diet appeared to attenuate caught many researchers off guard. Clearly, the diet was able to shift metabolism and genetic expression at some base level that prevented, rejuvenated, and protected cells, tissues, and organs (notably the brain) from the accumulation of disease causing damage. Like epilepsy, in most cases the exact influence ketones were having on the variety of diseases remained elusive. Howland's question became vastly expanded.

The Charlie Foundation became a conduit for the ketogenic diet's sudden expansion in interest. The calls, once dominated by the pleas of epileptic patients, made an abrupt shift to other diseases. Now, around the turn of the century, when the phone rang, or an email came it, it was most likely a cancer patient, or someone with Alzheimer's, or Parkinson's, or other more obscure problems. The Foundation decided to evolve, and allowed itself to be led be the science. They changed their name from The *Charlie Foundation for pediatric epilepsy* to The *Charlie Foundation for ketogenic therapies*.

Suddenly Zupec-Kania found herself teaching the diet to a vastly expanded group of health professionals. "We get more calls from cancer patients than epileptics now," she said. Zupec-Kania has noticed the utility of the diet continues to heave and undulate, covering additional ailments; its circle of effectiveness, surprisingly, continues to expand. "I'm getting more and more calls from people with migraines which 16% of Americans suffer from. We've found out the diet is super effective for migraines. And surprisingly, the other one is hot flashes from menopause. The ketogenic diet, even a liberal ketogenic diet, cures hot flashes."

For most of history epilepsy was viewed as a supernatural possession. Even today, vestiges of a mystical dimension linger. We know the disease is biological in origin, but it remains an enigma, it transcends our ability to succinctly explain it. That a subtle shift in energy metabolism is able to exorcise epileptic fits evokes imagery of preternatural healing; a biological force beyond our understanding. Incredibly, the discovery that the beneficial transition to ketone metabolism extends far past epilepsy, into unimaginable arenas of disease, only carries this image further – as evocative as it is astonishing.

The literature reflects this feeling; words like "magical, superfuel, jet-fuel, and magic bullet," slip from the pens of typically skeptical, objective and clinical scientists. The turn of the century marked the transition. The door is now open to a new era of medicine that, refreshingly, might have more to do with prevention than the never-ending cat and mouse game of diagnosing and treating disease after they have become intractably embedded – a game that is almost by definition, impossible to win. But it even goes beyond prevention. Ketone research has seduced us into imagining it might be possible to lift ourselves onto even higher planes of health and vitality. A bold new era of medicine beckons. Never have we asked if our health can be elevated, optimized, and extended with such vast technological resources at our fingertips.

The hybrid nature of human metabolism to utilize ketones as an energy source was not fully appreciated until the 1960's. And even then it was typically confused with diabetic ketoacidosis – a pathological condition that has nothing to do with fasting or nutritional ketosis in general. Nevertheless the two were lumped together and the true disease modifying potential of nutritional ketosis was not fully appreciated until around the turn of the century. We now know, the shift to ketone metabolism goes far beyond the swapping of one fuel for another. Hidden just below the surface we've uncovered a new layer of complexity: we now know ketones are absolutely profound in their impact to human physiology. Critically, they act as signaling molecules and carry deeply conserved messages to our DNA – messages that vastly impact our overall health.

Ketones change the architecture of our DNA, rearranging the way it is expressed, turning on the same rejuvenating pathways stimulated by caloric restriction or periodic fasting. Ketones appear to powerfully reduce inflammatory pathways – the smoldering process that is blamed for a vast spectrum of problems, even a reduction of overall lifespan. There is a growing consensus that most of the so called modern disease of civilization

– obesity, type 2 diabetes, and Alzheimer's (now called type 3 diabetes), cancer and many others – all ripple outward from a central core of metabolic dysfunction. These modern diseases, once considered pathologically distinct, converge to the same central place – a place that ketone metabolism concentrates its profoundly rejuvenating and repairing capacity. As Dr. Veech has said, "Ketosis is a normal physiological state. I would argue it is the normal state of man. It's not normal to have a McDonald's and a Delicatessen on every corner. It's normal to starve." Perhaps many of our modern ailments are a result of stepping too far from our natural state of existence.

It's easy to recognize the societal resistance to any rigid dietary adjustment and the search is underway to find shortcuts. "The 20th century was about understanding the ketogenic diet," said Dr. Wheless. "The 21st century is going to be about trying to capture its incredible benefits in a pill."

Science is a building that is constantly under construction. The progress we are making today rises from a foundation built by others. In addition to all those mentioned in the article, the work of Drs. Richard Veech, Sami Hashim and Henri Brunengraber has laid the concrete that we in this field all work and build. These metabolic gurus were responsible for opening the blinds and illuminating the therapeutic potential of exogenous ketone supplementation.

Standing on the shoulders of these giants, our laboratory at University of South Florida has been studying the effects of ketone supplementation on numerous disease states, physical performance and resilience against extreme environments. Could these small molecules – once thought to be metabolic waste – hold the potential to treat and prevent a constellation of metabolic related illness? Do they capture the time honored benefits of caloric restriction or intermittent fasting? Can they enhance our health, vitality and longevity – allowing the baby boomers, a generation that refuses to *go gently into that good night*, to extract more from life for longer? The initial results look promising.The data emerging rapidly from studies on nutritional ketosis are compelling and have far reaching implications. Perhaps Jim Abrahams said it best: "The genie is out of the bottle."

Acknowledgements
Thanks to the authors for their kind permission to publish these texts:

- **Dr. Thomas Seyfried,** Boston College

His website: https://tomseyfried.com/

His book at Amazon:
https://www.amazon.com/Cancer-Metabolic-Disease-Management-Prevention/dp/0470584920

- **Dr. Dominic D'Agostino**

His website: https://www.ketonutrition.org/

- **Travis Christofferson, M.S.**

His foundation to support Dr. Seyfrieds Research:
https://foundationformetaboliccancertherapies.com/

His books at Amazon:
https://www.amazon.com/Travis-Christofferson/e/B00OAOSZOA

- **Julie Foucher, M.D.**

Her website: https://pursuing-health.com/

We also thank **CrossFit** for hosting the talks and their support!

Their website: https://www.crossfit.com/

Last, but not least: We would also like to thank **Robb Wolf** for his outstanding work and insightful platform,

His website: https://robbwolf.com/

Sources

Chapter

1) Text (editors revised transcription) and slides based on Youtube video:

Channel: „ CrossFit® "

Channel-Url:

https://www.youtube.com/channel/UCtcQ6TPwXAYgZ1Mcl3M1vng

Title: " Dr. Thomas Seyfried: Cancer as a Mitochondrial Metabolic Disease "

Video-Url: https://www.youtube.com/watch?v=KusaU2taxow

2) Text (editors revised transcription) and slides based on Youtube video:

Channel: „ CrossFit® "

Channel-Url:

https://www.youtube.com/channel/UCtcQ6TPwXAYgZ1Mcl3M1vng

Title: " Dr. Dominic D'Agostino: Emerging Applications of Nutritional Ketosis "

Video-Url: https://www.youtube.com/watch?v=_blupWpZ5F4

(Minute 32-43 / 54-57)

3) Text (editors revised transcription) based on Youtube video:

Channel: „ Julie Foucher "

Channel-Url:

https://www.youtube.com/channel/UCWDto2R36n9pwwXq1HgjYHA

Title: " Challenging Conventional Cancer Care with Dr. Thomas Seyfried - PH97 "

Video-Url: https://www.youtube.com/watch?v=_beGwmBYBlo

4)   **Article:** Taken from https://robbwolf.com/

Article URL:
https://robbwolf.com/2015/09/24/the-origin-and-future-of-the-ketogenic-diet-part-1/ (and following)

Article Title: „ The Origin (and future) of the Ketogenic Diet "

Article authors: Dr. Dominic D'Agostino & Travis Christofferson

Made in the USA
Las Vegas, NV
01 October 2023

78369338R00075